ANIMAL
HEALING

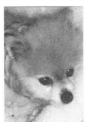

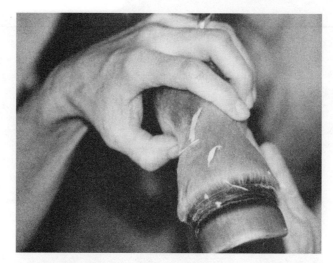

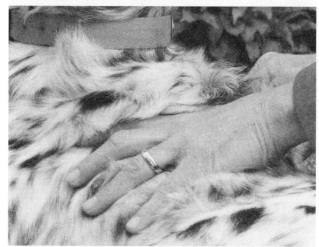

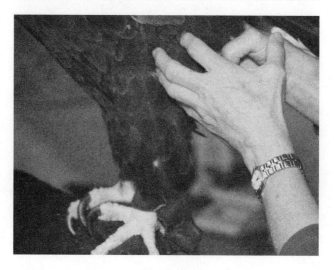

ANIMAL HEALING

The Power of Rolfing®

STRUCTURAL INTEGRATION

Briah Anson

MILL CITY PRESS ▶ MINNEAPOLIS 2011

Mill City Press, Inc.
212 Third Avenue North, Suite 290
Minneapolis, Minnesota 55401
612-455-2294
www.millcitypublishing.com

ISBN: 978-1-936400-97-3
LCCN: 2010943141

Printed in the United States of America

Book design and composition: Judy Gilats

Front cover art: Briah Anson

Front cover photograph: Peter Koeleman

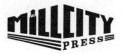

I DEDICATE THIS BOOK
to the memory
of Mac who saved my father's life
and to all our animal friends
who so willingly show us
their unconditional love.
With deep appreciation!

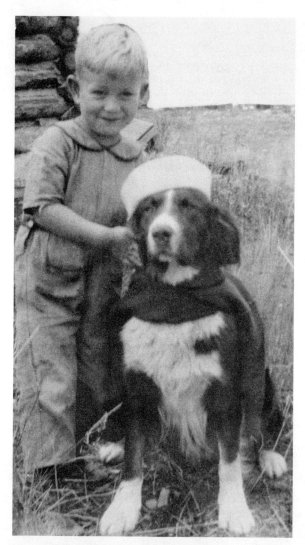

True Buddies in Life! This photo kindled my heart and represents my connection to the possibilities and importance of our animals being truly our kindred spirits.

My Dad and Mac

My dad grew up in Wisdom, Montana, which was rugged ranch land in the 1920s. When he was four years old he and his six-year-old sister, Helen, strayed away from home with their dog, Mac, who was a large collie/shepherd mix. Drawn to a good-sized canal that was flowing quite fast due to the early spring snow melt from the mountains, my dad ventured to the edge of the canal, which had a deep drop off. The ground gave in and he slipped into the water. Mac instantly went to the edge and grabbed him by his suspenders and held his head above the water.

Helen ran the long block back to the house and told my grandmother that Bobby had drowned. Needless to say, my grandmother took off running to the site and found Mac still holding my dad by the suspenders with his head above water. She fished him out; his life had clearly been saved by Mac.

A few months later there would be another incident that demonstrated Mac's rescue abilities. My grandmother had put my dad out to play in the yard; she tied one end of a rope firmly around his waist and tied the other end to the house to prevent another life and death mishap. My dad's exploring and pioneering ways started very early. He managed to free himself from the house and took off running down the middle of the street. Mac took off after him, grabbed the end of the rope, and pulled him back home. Once again, Mac saved my dad from imminent danger.

Contents

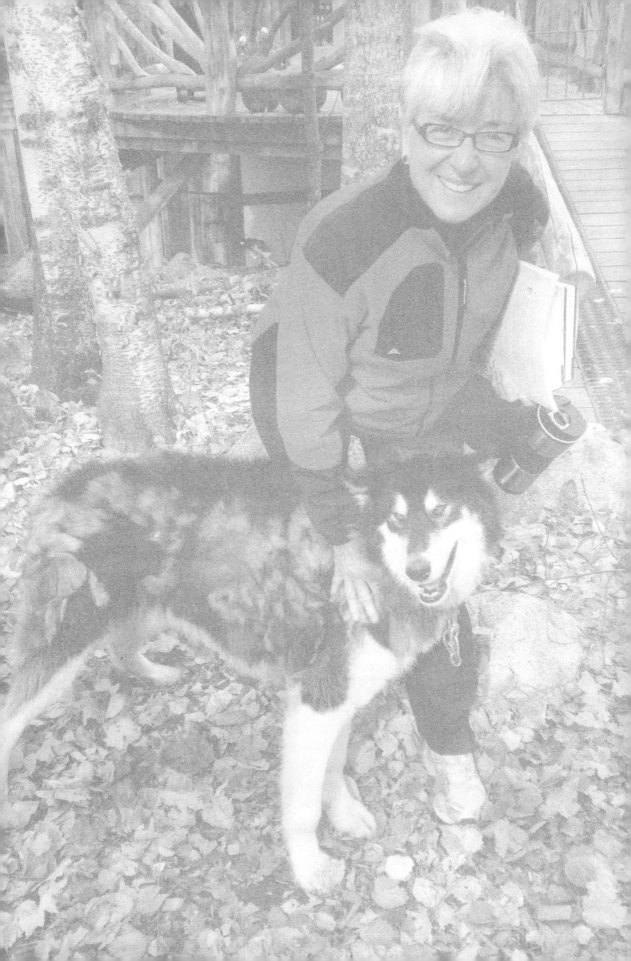

Foreword

PAUL SCHURKE, *Director of Wintergreen Dogsled Lodge and Arctic Adventures, and North Pole explorer*

If you enjoy animal stories as much as I do, you're in for a great read. In most books about animals (especially my childhood favorite, James Herriot's "All Creatures Great and Small"), they're always getting in and out of mischief. But in this delightful book, a very uplifting one, they're getting healed! You'll witness the health and happiness of these animals being transformed through the hands and heart of Briah Anson and her passionate application of Rolfing® Structural Integration (SI).

Since Rolfing was developed fifty years ago, it has helped reverse the effects of trauma, from illness and injury to the everyday impacts of gravity for thousands of people. Rolfers™ like Briah stretch and apply pressure to fascia, our connective tissue, to restore alignment in the body and to help correct aches and pains, restricted mobility, and poor posture. Rolfers have found that fascial adhesions in one part of the body can cause problems elsewhere. Like a knit sweater, pulling or sticking in one area of fascia or muscle may cause tissue distortions in another area. Correcting tissue imbalance becomes a holistic treatment.

During the first few months of her Rolfing career, which began in 1979, Briah wondered if these same benefits could extend to animals. That hunch came naturally to her given her childhood affinity for animals. When her first efforts (a lame thoroughbred mare named Petey) transformed this misaligned horse to a regal one with stately conformation, she knew she was onto something. And she has been Rolfing animals ever since, as you'll learn in this compilation of some three dozen case studies about animals (both wild and domestic) who've benefited from Briah's Rolfing skills.

It's an incredible menagerie: cats, dogs and horses, as well as guinea pigs, llamas, eagles, an owl, a rooster, a cougar and, perhaps most intriguing of all, an up close and personal encounter with a wild moose named Mike. Adding to the book's novelty are the various perspectives from which the stories are told. Some are told by Briah, some by the animals' owners and some are a dialogue between the two, which is appropriate since most of these pets were treated at the request of owners who'd benefited from Rolfing SI themselves.

All the stories are endearing. You'll meet Tita, a rottweiler pup who suffered from such severe hip problems that her owners feared they might have to put her down. Following Rolfing sessions, Tita was bounding up and down stairs, grew into a healthy dog, and lived a long full life. You'll meet Cinnabar, a golden eagle whose wing had been crippled by a gunshot wound. His flight ability improved dramatically following Rolfing sessions and Cinnabar was able to soar. And there's Rufus, the great horned owl, who suffered a dislocated jaw when hit by a car. The benefits of Rolfing became apparent as he was able once again to tear and eat his prey.

Briah credits her ability to her instinctive understanding of the anatomy of form. For example, she views four-legged animals as having two sets of vertical lines. She palpates them to determine tissue imbalances and then, through the Rolfing process, aligns their energy from the ground up through the legs to the shoulders or pelvis. Then she envisions the midline up through the torso, neck and head as she seeks to harmonize the animal's posture and movement. "It really becomes a sculpting process," she says.

Does that mean Rolfing SI is more art than science? Not according to Dr. Julie Wilson, Associate Professor of Veterinary Medicine at the University of Minnesota. As outlined in the book, she collaborated with Briah on the treatment for Indy, a foal with a severe congenital defect that prevented it from standing and nursing. Briah began to work on him when he was just three days old. The results? Briah's help "really made a difference," said Dr. Wilson. "This was my first experience with Rolfing as an adjunctive therapy and my clinical impression was that the results were more sustainable, and absolutely progressive over the three visits."

Rolfing SI is science and art coming together. That's a powerful combination, especially when extreme treatment measures are needed. Bodies pushed to their limits sustain tremendous wear and tear. That's as true for animal athletes as for human ones. That was my connection to Briah and the benefits of Rolfing SI. My family's livelihood and lifestyle is built around dogsledding. Our kennel of canine athletes is the key to our lifestyle here at Wintergreen Dogsled Lodge in Minnesota's North Woods. Our pure-bred Canadian Inuit dogs live to pull. The power of that instinct is truly awe-inspiring, but it can take a toll on their physical well-being.

Our chance encounter with Briah occurred just after Thistle, one of our beloved sled dogs, had suddenly lost control of his hindquarters. The frantic look in his eyes spoke of his tremendous pain and tore at our heart strings. When steroids proved ineffective, the vet advised that we put him down. But we weren't prepared to give up and neither was Thistle. With marvelous serendipity, Briah happened into our lives just then and immediately applied her skills to Thistle. As you'll read in this book, a bit of magic has since transpired.

Here at Wintergreen, we enjoy a collateral benefit of Briah's visits. We've learned from her therapy on our animals just how much they enjoy being handled. While we don't have the skills to do Rolfing SI on them ourselves, we're all much more inclined to spend time massaging them now. As we knead their powerful chest and back muscles and they respond by leaning into us and sighing with eyes nearly closed, we can feel our bond with these canine teammates intensify.

I'm delighted that Rolfing SI has helped bolster not only the health and happiness of our sled dogs, but our friendship and connection with them as well. In reading this book, you'll find that your own passion for animals and your relationships with them will also be enhanced. And you'll learn more about a system of transformation that may enhance the quality of life for both you and your pets.

Paul Schurke
Ely, Minnesota
NOVEMBER, 2010

What is Rolfing® Structural Integration?

"When the tone of the soft tissue is balanced, there is a sensation of lightness in the body." DR. IDA P. ROLF

Rolfing® Structural Integration was developed over sixty years ago by a remarkable biochemist and physiologist, Dr. Ida P. Rolf. Her many years of research and practice brought her to an understanding that all physical bodies, at all times, must deal with the effects of gravity. The purpose of Rolfing SI is to better balance the physical body around a vertical line in the field of gravity so that gravity begins to support the body, rather than tear it down. The "organ" of response to the gravitational field is the myofascial system.

Both human and animal bodies have a myofascial system. The myofascial system encapsulates, envelops, attaches, supports and relates all body components. It is a highly adaptive and plastic system. It accounts for a considerable proportion of the body's outward form. Its properties of elasticity and plasticity, and the ability to hold a shape are what make physical changes possible and permanent.

Disorder in the myofascial system can result from physical and emotional trauma; infection and disease processes; poor habits of posture and movement; stress; the biomechanical wear and tear of everyday living; and compensations in the structure from any of the preceding problems. This disorder causes a deterioration of tonal balance, appropriate density, necessary resiliency and overall organization of the entire myofascial system.

More specifically, the myofascial system reacts to these disorders by shortening, thickening, twisting, binding, and gluing down the sheets, planes, and membranous layers of connective tissue. Physiological changes occur as the body modifies its myofascial environment to cope with new strain patterns.

Because the myofascial system is just that, a system, specific local distortions/injuries, etc. can cause a complex of changes in the whole system. Because we move as a whole, each restriction will soon modify the whole. Without skilled intervention, the myofascial system tends to become more "disintegrated" over time rather than more integrated.

Physical injuries and chronic emotional states contribute to shortening and thickening of connective tissue. They prevent the body from regaining its flow and freedom of movement. Thickening in one part of the body causes other parts to compensate.

Rolfing Structural Integration is a way of reversing this process. It is a series of ten sessions (with human clients, and varies in actual clock time depending on the scope of the work and the problems present) during which the Rolfer™ uses physical pressure (direct energy) to stretch and guide fascia to a place of easier movement. The Rolfer uses the plasticity and mobility of the myofascial system to balance, organize and align the body. Rolfing SI calls forth, through these highly skilled manipulations, appropriate organization, i.e., anatomically normal alignment and biomechanically efficient movement. In doing this, the major segments of the structure are brought toward their optimal arrangement in the gravitational field.

As myofascial restrictions are released, movement becomes more co-ordinated and refined. The body feels light, roomy and at ease. Flexibility, range of motion and joint stability all improve. The system is better able to handle stress of all kinds more effectively and easily. Reactive mechanical patterns of behavior are reduced or eliminated entirely. In summary, there is a distinct improvement in the operational soundness and efficiency in many, if not all, systems in the body. By restoring systemic balance, all functions improve.

Rolfing SI is primarily an educational and restorational method which often has profoundly therapeutic results. The primary goal is the establishment and restoration of balance in the body. In this process the reduction of symptoms occurs, often very dramatically. The paradox is that this occurs by focusing on balance rather than symptom reduction. This differentiates Rolfing SI from most other methods of working with the physical body.

Rolfing SI balances the fascial network by taking advantage of its ability to hold a shape induced by applied pressure. In a carefully developed sequence, the Rolfer reverses randomizing influences from the environment, moving tissue toward symmetry and balance that is called for so clearly by the architecture of the body.

A key principle is that "the body is a plastic medium." The most immediate plastic component of the body that we can get our hands on, and physically alter in form and function, is fascia. Fascia gives form to the body; it is the most pervasive tissue.

Fascia surrounds every muscle cell, controlling and guiding its function. It is a continuous wrapping that envelopes all the muscle tissue in the body, as well as every bone, nerve, organ, ligament, joint, cartilage and vessel. Fascia can be broken down into three anatomical divisions:

- ▶ Superficial fascia which is below the skin.
- ▶ Deep fascia, around muscle, bone, nerves, vessels and organs.
- ▶ Deepest fascia, the dura of the craniosacral system.

Fascia, from the Latin word meaning bands, responds to trauma by tightening and shortening, creating a chain reaction with other parts of the body and, over time, pulling the body out of proper alignment.

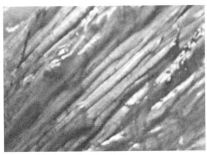

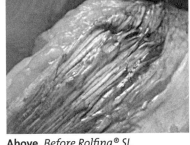

Above. *Before Rolfing® SI.*
Below. *After Rolfing® SI.*

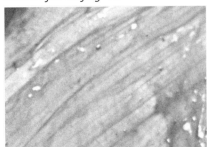

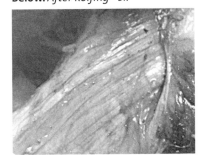

Bovine fascia from a lower leg muscle (gastrocnemius) before and after manipulation shows how tight fibrous connective tissue can be loosened with manual therapies such as Rolfing® SI. Photos courtesy of Stephen Evanko.

Dr. Rolf's vision of initiating or restoring structural and functional balance is what aids the individual person or animal to achieve their maximum potential and birthright: a body that uses gravity efficiently, effectively and appropriately. As the Rolfer facilitates the release of outmoded and debilitating patterns in the structure, the order brought about in the structure provides an environment in which a form of healing occurs quite naturally. This is facilitated by the return to the anatomical blueprint of the body, resulting in peace and order in the myofascial system.

Rolfing SI seeks to illuminate the integrative and unifying qualities that characterize the nature of whole systems. It is very exciting and inspiring to see more minds turning to the exploration of the wonders which the body, in the brilliant wisdom of its design, already knows.

Adapting the Human 10-series to Animal Work

"Lines in a body are not mystical structures;
they are where forces balance." DR. IDA P. ROLF

Learning to watch and understand movement is key to a good Rolfing series, whether human or animal. Getting a thorough look at an animal's motion is my first task. With a horse, for instance, I want to see how the compensations in the structure are organizing themselves through the whole body. I look at the proportions of each of the segments—how the head fits the neck, how the neck hooks onto the shoulders, where the front legs are positioned under the shoulders, and if there is a torque anywhere.

Then I try mentally to draw straight lines through the horse and see where they bend. Is there a line through the body of the horse, or is it sagging? Can I draw a midline through the trunk of the horse and up through the neck? From the side, can I see two sets of vertical lines from the ground, through the legs and into the pelvis or shoulder? When I watch the horse move toward me I want to be able to draw a vertical plane through the center of the head and straight back. When I watch the horse move away from me I look to see if one side of the pelvis is higher, if it is torqued to one side, how the legs track, and if there is support coming up from the ground.

I watch all four legs in movement and the spacing of the legs as the horse pushes off. Can he come through his legs? Can he push from the hind end? Is there movement through to the head? Is there effort in the gait or is there ease? Is there dynamic motion that looks light or is there density and harshness? What sound do his hooves make hitting the ground?

One of the principles of Rolfing SI is to align the structure in gravity. What does this mean for a quadruped? A four-legged creature has two sets of vertical lines coming up from the ground. A structure with a healthy relationship with gravity would present with balance in the spacing of their segments. There would be a symmetry and evenness of tissue tone from side to side, top to bottom, and front to back. In movement, each segment should be able to extend and lengthen through space. There will be a visible transmission of movement through the segments that looks open and fluid.

After I've observed everything I can about the animal I then move on to the hands-on work. I always start with opening up the respiration of the body. In a four-legged it's essential to start by freeing up the shoulder girdle. Then I work back through the body to free up the pelvis, and then some organizing work to free up the neck and the head.

Depending on the size and density of the animal, I generally work from surface to deep. I feel the condition of the tissues in their different layers, and work with wherever I feel non-resilient tissue. I feel for a lack of motion in the fascia, and for tissues that are not well-hydrated.

Balance is the primary goal of the work, and by this I mean an equal tissue tone from front to back, between the two sides, and between the top and bottom halves of the body. There's another type of balance as well: the balance between the deeper layers of fascia closest to the bone and the superficial fascia. But this is not simple tissue work that I am doing, it is Rolfing Structural Integration, with all that implies. I resist the urge to work on presenting symptoms (even though the owner is probably fretting about it), because this is not the Rolfing premise that makes it different and effective. This organ of structure, fascia, is a very resilient, elastic, and plastic medium. It is interconnected from the cranium out through the tail. I'm not done until I see flow, grace, and ease in their movement.

Once the practitioner understands the relationship between balance, alignment, and movement, (s)he then just keeps "circling the wagons" until (s)he gets that to come about. All lines of transmission going through the structure need to be addressed in a sequential, organized process. This is easy to make sense of once a practitioner has truly understood the goals of the classical 10-series, originally discovered by Dr. Rolf. I am creatively applying the 10-series to animals ranging from a small bird to a large horse by understanding and addressing the goals of each of the sessions, whether I do one or ten sessions.

The number of sessions that I do with each species of animal depends on the size of the animal and the issues it is carrying in its structure. I typically spend about an hour as the format for scheduling sessions. With all animals, I work slowly so that the animal can track the changes through its structure and nervous system. It is always a cooperative venture between myself and the animal client. Establishing that cooperative connection is essential, and I work slowly so that layer by layer, the animal can integrate the information and the changes.

In working this way I have found that I can efficiently build up tissue, and allow the animal time to grow into more of who they truly are. Since I began my practice as a Rolfer™ one of my guiding principles in understanding this Rolfing work is that I am working to evoke the true essence of who lives inside. The stories in this book are a sampling of my experiences with the animal clients that I have had over the years. They represent a wide cross section of the issues that bring these clients in the door, and the unexpected results that arise long after the sessions are finished. Their owners have often been surprised at the multi-dimensional changes they have witnessed from even one or two Rolfing sessions with their animals.

Briah's Story

I've often said to people that in my life I bonded with dogs and animals first.

I was born in Costa Rica, the oldest of three children. From very early on I had a deep love for animals. I still have photographs and memories of my first year and a half, being in a playpen with my two black cocker spaniels, Sally and Susie. After the cocker spaniels, we had a couple of boxers, and some of the photographs show me sleeping downstairs on the floor cuddled up with them. We had a bird in the house and a cat. When I was around eight years old I dreamed of owning a horse. When we moved out to the country I saved my allowance for a year and bought my first horse. It was kind of funny—it was half horse and half mule and it was pretty pathetic looking, but it was mine. Then there came the saving of more allowances and buying more horses, and so my history has always been with animals.

By the time I left Costa Rica when I was close to eighteen, I'd already owned half a dozen horses. We lived up in the foothills of the mountains in the town of Escazu which was not an expensive place to have horses. We had big pastures surrounding our house that were never used, so that's where I did a lot of my riding. There were also dirt roads that went far up into the hills and mountains that provided me with ample places to ride and a lot of great fun. I remember people in Costa Rica say-

My primal bonding with my cocker spaniel Sally, age five months

ing that I had *caballos con mucho brio*—horses with great spirit—and that became the genesis of my first name, Briah, after I became a Rolfing® Structural Integrator. I've always had this tremendous love for horses and dogs—those were the animals that I primarily bonded with.

When I came to the United States, I thought my life would take the route of becoming a professional golfer, but I went to college instead and became interested in subjects like psychology, philosophy, and religion. My last two years of college were spent at a very special school in Michigan called Oakland University. I became involved in student activities and was a student delegate to the Board of Trustees. After graduating, I developed a passion for this kind of work and went on to get my Masters in Counseling and Student Personnel work.

I followed this detour for a number of years working as an Assistant Coordinator for Residence Halls at Penn State while I earned my Masters degree. This path took me to Colorado College where I was the Dean of Women's Housing, then on to the University of Minnesota Morris, to take up an opportunity to build an amazing Residential Life program. I was there for five years pondering whether to get my doctorate, but I kept feeling that there was something else brewing inside of me and I wasn't sure what that was.

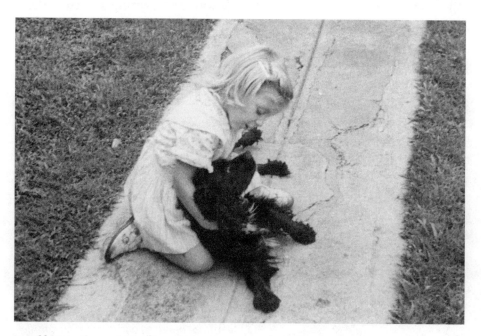

A Rolfer™ in the making. (Age 2)

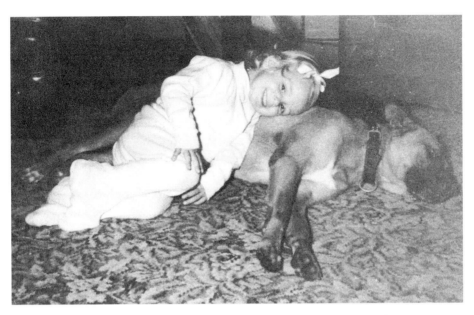

My early comfort with animals. My favorite place to sleep … with Bo. (Age 2 years 8 months.)

I decided to take a month off and go to a thirty-day psychotherapy intensive in Estes Park, Colorado. This workshop was led by Anne Wilson Schaef who is a process psychotherapist. There were eighteen psychologists from around the country as well as some seminary students from Yale. We lived and ate there, doing our own personal work about twelve hours a day.

It was about the third day into this workshop that I had my first deep body massage. I was getting about two of these a week and they had a profound impact on me, releasing a lot of my own life history. During the second week of this workshop as I was doing my Buddhist chanting, it came to me that I should become a Rolfer™.

I had heard of Rolfing® SI five years earlier at an encounter group leadership workshop in La Jolla with Carl Rogers. I was very taken with how one of the trainers presented and carried herself—she had a very regal presence. I had the great fortune to ride to the airport with her, and out of the blue she starting talking about her experience with the Rolfing process. It was probably the most significant personal growth adventure she had ever taken. She talked so much about the connection of the mind and body, and how all of our history is embedded in the body, that it made quite an impression on me. I had started practicing Buddhism just that year, and what she said reverberated closely with my new practice.

Five years later, I attended another thirty-day intensive, this one a lot more intrapsychic, and doing my own life unearthing. In the second week of this workshop, I was chanting and it came to me that Rolfing SI was what I was to do. I went back to the group and announced this. All I really knew about it was what that one woman had said to me five years earlier, but with the deep tissue massage I was now getting I was experiencing first hand the profound impact that deep tissue work has in releasing the intrapsychic. It was more available to process in my work with Anne Schaef and in that group situation. I felt that in one month I had grown by ten years. I felt that all my education in psychology and counseling, the different workshops I'd attended, and my internship at Penn State, had coalesced in this very rich and profound month. I knew there was a different direction my life was calling out for—it was time to take all of this education and point it down a new path.

I proceeded to drive to the closest Rolfer™ every Saturday, which was 300 miles roundtrip to Minneapolis. I remember that my Rolfer, Judith Mayanja, was surprised and wondered how I could know that I wanted to be a Rolfer without having first experienced it. But I felt that it was in my body, it was literally bone-deep within me, and the experience of going through the sessions revealed that this was exactly what I wanted to do.

I had grown up in Costa Rica being extremely athletic. We lived right next to a country club and that was my playground. I learned how to play golf and tennis at the age of eight and competed nationally in those sports, as well as in swimming. I had also started taking ballet two to three times a week when I was eight years old, and performing in the national theater in Costa Rica. Using my body as an expression of myself was very important. I remember even as I grew up, how important it was for me to have good style, and I worked very, very hard. I took many lessons in all these sports, not because it was important for me to win, but rather to have a good swing, a good stroke, to ride beautifully. I have always had a very natural swing and I was a natural athlete, but I appreciated people that also carried out the sport in an aesthetic, beautiful way. So I think that part of the genesis of my coming to this Rolfing work had already been birthed long before I made what felt like a decision out of the blue. It had been growing organically for many, many years.

I now understood that people carried their histories in their bodies and that without work like Rolfing SI those histories would stay locked inside and thwart people from fulfilling the potentials they'd been born with. The goal of this work is to align the body in the field of gravity, to establish balance in all of the tendons, ligaments, muscles, and connective tissues; from the outside of the body to the inside; from the front to the back; from top to bottom—to establish a sense of order and balance that are critical to a body being able to work well, perform well, and prevent injuries that come from misalignments. A body of this type would facilitate healing very quickly. These concepts, as I started reading and studying about the Rolfing process, all made complete sense to me.

When I moved to the United States, my godmother in Grosse Pointe, Michigan, took me to volunteer with physically and mentally handicapped children. I remember that being one of the most challenging experiences of my life. I remember how frustrating it was to help these children eat or do activities that we wouldn't think twice about, and it would take a lot of time. I remember visualizing being able to sculpt these children's bodies and seeing them functional, seeing them working well. I think that experience was at the root of my becoming a Rolfer™ as well.

I went on to the Rolf Institute® of Structural Integration and completed all my studies in May of 1979, returning to Minneapolis where I had promised about ten people that I would take them through the Rolfing process. I did two sessions a week with each of them because I had decided to move to Kansas City, Missouri.

In July I opened up my Rolfing practice in Kansas City, and one of my very first clients was a man by the name of Fred Kahn, an equestrian and teacher of horseback riding and jumping. He could see how much the Rolfing series was helping his alignment and one day he mentioned that his thoroughbred hunter-jumper horse had sustained an injury. She had become lame, the vets had not been able to do anything, and he had a national competition coming up. He wanted me to work on his mare, Petey, and see what could happen.

I told Fred that I had never done Rolfing® SI on a horse, but I was sure that I could figure this out. Mind you, I had a poodle at home named Kore that I immediately did sessions on when I returned from my training, and I had quickly ascertained that animal tissue is animal tissue, whether in a human or a four-legged or winged creature. I had already worked on two or three dogs and didn't see any reason why I couldn't figure out how to do this with a horse. I was probably one of the earliest pioneers of doing Rolfing work with animals so there was no one to teach me. Having had horses and ridden them, and having an eye for Rolfing work, I quickly figured out that in a four-legged creature there are two sets of vertical lines—one going up through the front legs into the shoulder; another one going up through the hind legs and into the hind quarters. Then there is a midline that goes through the length of the body; and one up through the neck and head.

Just as with humans, there is a Rolfing SI template. There are goals for every session in the sequence of ten we use for organizing a person, but what evolved from my first horse-Rolfing experience with Petey was a five-session approach. In these five sessions I worked on the horse for a couple of hours each time, and spaced the sessions about a week apart. This turned out to be an adequate number of sessions for Petey to take on a healthy alignment with gravity. Because horses and other animals do not have all the mental/emotional baggage that we do as humans, and they are much more primal in terms of their connection in their nervous systems, this kind of work can be accomplished more quickly.

There is a story in my earlier book about Petey with before and after photographs, and you cannot even tell that it's the same horse. One horse looks like a misaligned old animal, and the other one is a gorgeous horse with the most beautiful conformation.

Following this experience with Fred's horse, I worked with several of his clients' horses. Soon I was invited to work on my clients' ailing or aging dogs and cats. So it started growing, and pretty soon I was doing Rolfing sessions with birds, which led to an invitation to rehab a Golden Eagle, and then an owl that had been run over by a car. You can read the stories of these animals and many more, like the cougar and Mike the Moose, in the following chapters.

I shared my experiences with my instructors at the Rolf Institute®, some of whom were enthusiastic, but for the most part I suspect that most Rolfers back then were a little worried by it. Rolfing SI was not well known and it was felt that this use of the work might skew the public's perception of it in a negative way. Consequently, I was not very proactive about publicizing this kind of work with animals. But, I loved it! The results I got with the rehab work were very quick and that became my entry point into working with animals. I've been doing Rolfing Structural Integration with people and animals now for thirty years. For the most part, the animals I've worked with have belonged to clients or their friends.

The Benefits of Rolfing SI for Animals

Rolfing Structural Integration was popularized in the mid-1960s as a treatment for human ailments, and as a great innovation in the human potential movement. In the last twenty years, Rolfing SI has begun to cross over into the animal kingdom, primarily because pet owners experience the work themselves and then look for alternatives when they hit a dead end with traditional veterinary options. Any animal suffering from movement limitations that result from injury, disease, surgical trauma and even old age may benefit from Rolfing sessions. Cats that no longer leap to their favorite counter, dogs that compete a bit too enthusiastically in agility competitions or field trials; horses recovering from lameness, colic surgery, or founder; and birds with injured wings are some examples.

Rolfing SI has also been known to aid in the recovery from secondary or tertiary responses to trauma—the muscle spasms, soreness and compensatory patterns that linger long after the wounds heal. Practitioners and clients also sing the praises of this work for correcting behavior problems associated with certain traumas or even abuse.

Rolfing SI has begun to cross over into the animal kingdom, primarily because pet owners experience the work themselves and then look for alternatives when they hit a dead end with traditional veterinary options.

Owners and trainers of performance horses and dogs find Rolfing SI especially useful as both a remedy for the aches and strains that inevitably accompany athletics, and as a tune-up strategy to keep them primed for competition. Mary Agneessens, who has taught an equine Rolfing process in Arizona and Kentucky with me, has said that horse races can be won by a nose, by a half inch. "If a horse is sore or fatigued somewhere, or doesn't run straight, that could be your half an inch. Rolfing isn't going to make them faster, it's not going to take a horse that can't run and give him the ability to run, but it is going to take a horse with some ability and help fulfill its potential."

With sporting athletes, as part of their athletic training, Rolfing SI keeps them agile, pliable and athletic. Mary Agneessens claims that it's good for an animal's ego, that it's a real confidence booster. "If they believe in themselves, it's amazing what they will do. Horses will win races simply because they believe they can. I work on helping them maintain their own personal space so they know where they are in space and have a sense of who they are inside. If you have three horses running down a stretch, it's the horse that doesn't give up his space that wins."

But it's the day in, day out, constant training for the show ring, the hunt field, or the racetrack, that most often calls the Rolfer out for treating what Michael Reams, another horse Rolfer, terms "the microtraumas of training: the results of ill-fitting tack, heavy shoes, poor footing, a sloppy rider, and maybe just too much enthusiasm."

"Horses have the same problems as human athletes: tight hamstrings, sore muscles in their hind ends, back problems, hip problems, and neck problems," says Tessie Brungardt, Rolfing SI instructor. "*We* made it up that horses are for riding, horses didn't make that up."

Another Rolfer, Greg Wilder, agrees. "The equine structure did not evolve over millions of years to carry a hundred pounds right where we put a saddle. The instant we get on and begin to ride, we have overstressed the structure for what it's intended to do. Sixty-five percent of what I work on with horses comes from the saddle and rider, from carrying extra weight that they didn't evolve to carry."

Whatever horses may think about racing down the track, trotting a hundred mile endurance course or jumping seven-foot fences in the Olympics, practitioners say it's clear they just love the Rolfing work. "A horse almost sat on me," Agneessens said. "I was working on a place on his hind end and he started licking the handler, kissing the handler, and began to sit on my hand. It got funny. It looked like he was going to act like a dog and sit on my lap. When you hit the right spot, when you find the key, they just relax and lean into you."

A Typical Visit

If you're visiting a Rolfer for the first time, be prepared to give the practitioner a complete history of the animal, including the kind of work it does. For horses, jumping, racing, dressage, endurance. For dogs, obedience, agility, field trials. Include any surgery the animal has had, as well as accidents or traumas. Be sure to mention if there is something your animal has done in the past that it is not able to do now. You do not have to bring any medical records, x-rays, or referrals from your veterinarian.

The Rolfer will want to watch the animal move. For dogs and cats that usually just means letting the animal walk around for a few moments, on or off leash, while the Rolfer examines their gait, noting what moves and what doesn't. When I first work with an animal, I watch them lie down and get up, especially with older dogs. I watch where the motion seems to be hung up, and look at the curvature of the body through the barrel. The tail plays an important part in what is going on with the dog or the horse. The tail is part of the spine and many times it has a kink in it that you can't see, but you can feel as you manipulate it.

For horses, it's a little more complicated. Although the Rolfer will want to evaluate the horse's conformation and gaits without tack, owners should be prepared to tack up and ride so that the Rolfer can see if the saddle or rider is interfering with correct movement. In my experience working with horses, I look for symmetry in the movement of the legs, how motion flows through the whole body, and how the horse moves in straight lines or in ever-widening circles. Does he cross over correctly and equally in each direction when turning left and right, front and behind? Does he bend through the barrel equally in each direction? I pay particular attention to how all the parts connect. How the head connects to the neck, how the neck is related to the shoulders, how the legs move out of the shoulders, how the long body moves, how the hind end is hooked in, and how the legs come out of the hind end.

"Rolfing a four-legged animal is different from Rolfing a two-legged human being," says Mary Agneessens. "We try to teach people how to see equine movement, what's correct and what's not, what's a subtle sign of something compensating somewhere else. We work on how to approach the problem, how the nervous system of the horse operates, what the common strains are for the different ways the horse is used. For instance, if it is a racehorse, where do those problems arise? If it is a jumper, where do those problems arise? In a horse that is used for dressage, yet other issues arise. Having a background in horses is very beneficial in that you know what you're looking at. You know where things are functioning properly and where they are not, and I think that informs one's work as a Rolfer working with dogs or horses."

After the initial examination, the Rolfer, well, gets to work. Where I start depends on what part moves. The following stories tell the tales of what happens when movement returns.

The quotes were taken from "Rolf Your Pets," Norine Dworkin, *Natural Pet Magazine,* June 1996, vol. 5, no.3.

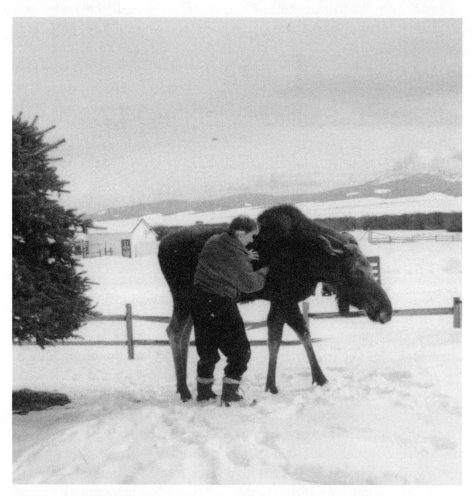

As I worked into his shoulder, Mike stretches down and out, cooperating with his own release. Photo by Marilyn Beech.

Mike the Moose from Montana

Briah recalls her experience in the Big Hole, Montana

I moved to Minnesota in July of 1998. I quickly rediscovered the wonders and beauty of the North Shore of Lake Superior and had some exciting moments seeing majestic moose on the side of the road grazing. The moose is a state icon in Minnesota and anyone who has any kind of encounter with one regards it as a fine event. It was then that I gave birth to the intention of doing a Rolfing® session on a moose. It occurred to me that I would gain a greater understanding of these Nordic people and their ways if I could find a moose to work on. I found myself announcing to people that somehow I was going to give a moose a Rolfing session. Each time I made this known, people would burst into laughter and proceed to tell me that that was just impossible. But I believed that working on a moose would help me more fully understand this Scandinavian land that felt so foreign to me.

Mind you, I had only moved 450 miles north from Kansas City, Missouri, to St. Paul, Minnesota, and yet the cultural background was very different than what I was accustomed to. I found people here to be emotionally held in and their physical structures mirrored this tradition. Expressing a range of emotion both positive and negative, the highs and lows, seemed to be more foreign to people in this Nordic land. I came to understand the lone introverted nature of the moose to be in rhythm with the Scandinavian temperament. I knew that I had moved to a place of educational, cultural and artistic excellence, to a land of hardworking determined people. However, I have always felt that the animal world functioned as my teacher to better understand the people with whom I worked.

I had no idea how I would find this moose. However, every kind of animal that I have done Rolfing sessions with came from my clear intention first to work with that particular species. Then through synchronicity it would come to pass.

A few months later, I was at my parent's home in Florida for Christmas and was looking through all the Christmas cards that my parents had received. I came upon a photo card of "Mike the Moose" drinking water out of a kitchen sink. I immediately thought to myself, "there's my moose." This moose lived on a 40,000-acre ranch in Wisdom, Montana, the birthplace of my father and the ranch of one of his best friends, Jack Hirschy.

I asked my parents to tell me about Mike and found out that Mike was an orphan that one of Jack's cowboys had found on the ranch. He'd brought the calf to Ann Hirschy to see if she could work her magic to keep this little one alive. She fed Mike and nursed him so that he would thrive, and they set him free to roam on their ranch. The Christmas photo of Mike had been taken when he was less than one year old. He would now be two years old.

My parents thought this was another of my ridiculous and dangerous ideas and just laughed it off. A month later, Jack and Ann Hirschy were visiting my folks from Montana to attend the Super Bowl. During their visit, my parents learned that Jack was having terrible back problems and was facing back surgery. My mother enthusiastically shared with Jack my book of Rolfing stories, *Rolfing®: Stories of Personal Empowerment,* which Jack read from cover to cover. He then proceeded to ask my mother if she would contact me to help them locate a Certified Rolfer™ who lived in his area.

This was my moment to seize. It just so happened that one of my best friends and Rolfing colleagues, Marilyn Beech, had moved from Kansas City to Missoula, Montana, which was only a two-and-a-half-hour drive from Wisdom. I proceeded to talk with Jack and propose to him that I would personally fly out to Montana from Minnesota and give him and Ann some free Rolfing sessions with the hope of being able to see Mike the Moose. Ann told me that Mike was over two years old which meant that his testosterone was elevated and he was getting quite wild. She also told me that they had very infrequent visits from Mike those days and that there was high probability of not seeing him at all. It mattered not to me. My desire was so strong that I intuitively thought that Mike and I would meet.

I arrived at their ranch close to dinnertime on March 5, 1999, which was my Dad's eightieth birthday. I was in his hometown of Wisdom.

There had been no sightings of Mike for weeks, and yet I had this incredibly jittery feeling that I would soon be meeting Mike. I had a couple of months to chant about this through my Buddhist practice. I felt that the encounter would be imminent as I had already connected with Mike spiritually.

When Marilyn and I arrived, Ann came out to greet us. She had been experiencing some troubling dizziness. I immediately went in to the house and set up the Rolfing table. I did a cranial session on Ann before dinner. Meals were in the cookhouse where all the cowboys and the Hirschy's ate their meals together.

With two feet of snow on the ground; it was still winter in Montana. Halfway through dinner I looked over to the window and saw this big animal walk by. It was Mike the Moose coming to meet me. Everyone was excited. The cook instantly gathered up leftovers for Mike to enjoy. They had built a four-foot-tall pole and nailed a large pan on top where Mike could feed. This was my opportunity. CARPE DIEM.

I followed Ann out since she had the connection with Mike. As he was hurriedly eating dinner, I stood next to Mike and started to do a little Rolfing SI on his left shoulder. One of my clients who was into Shamanic practices had given me the assignment of cutting a piece of moose mane for her medicine pouch. I whipped out my Swiss Army knife and cut a few locks of Mike's mane. I smelled his fur; it smelled clean and sweet. I figured I had better take him all in, not knowing if there would be another encounter.

As I was working, Mike suddenly stopped eating and raised his head up. The next thing I knew he had lunged about fifteen feet forward and gave a karate kick to a skunk that was in the process of climbing in the big pan of food scraps for the dog. He did this so quickly and precisely that the skunk never knew what hit him. This skunk did not even have time to spray us. We all thought that the skunk was dead. Mike quickly returned to his dinner and I noticed that my heart was beating a million miles an hour. I was processing how fast and ferocious this seemingly gentle creature had become. I knew then that one had better not mess with a moose. I suddenly appreciated all of the stories that people had told me about their fearful and healthy respect for this animal. I had seen a moose in action. He was fast and frighteningly precise.

A few minutes later we saw the skunk emerging out of the dog's pan and quickly staggering away. He wasn't dead after all. We were all amazed that the skunk never sprayed.

I returned to this impromptu Rolfing session and I noticed that Mike, even as he ate, was leaning into me just like the horses I'd worked on, so I knew that he was accepting this work. As he finished his food, he seemed to get a bit aggressive and I knew it was time to scoot back into the cookhouse. The next thing we knew, Mike was gone into the hills of the 40,000-acre ranch. It was all pretty exciting to me.

Breakfast was at 5:30 AM, which felt like an ungodly early time to eat. While we were having breakfast, Mike showed his face again at the window. I was no longer interested in breakfast. Ann and I went outside. Mike had his head down and seemed more feisty and aggressive than the previous day. In fact, he seemed interested in chasing us a bit and didn't seem to be too friendly. He sort of followed us, chasing us back to the house where we quickly disappeared.

I was feeling rather disappointed at that moment. Ann was cautioning me that Mike had reached the age where his behavior may be less predictable due to increased testosterone levels. Ann came up with the idea of getting some dried fruit as that was his favorite treat when he was younger. We went out with assorted fruit and Mike quickly and rather aggressively took it from us. Ann then said she thought we better call it quits for the day with the moose.

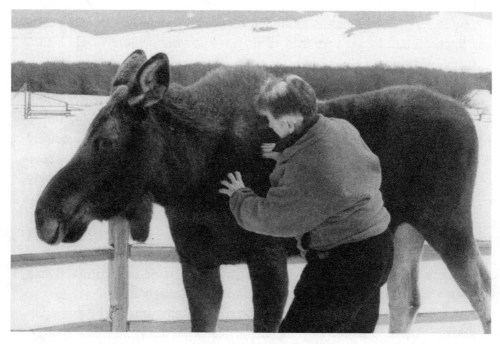

Mike returns for another session! Photo by Marilyn Beech.

I remember feeling disappointed that I might not have any more Rolfing SI encounters with Mike and just did not want to give up. I stood inside and looked out the window. I saw Mike standing outside. I remember thinking "What is he waiting for? More fruit?" After watching him I decided to quietly exit the house and see if I could make some contact with him. He just stood still as I stood next to him and once again I carefully and slowly started doing a little Rolfing SI on his left shoulder. He remained calm and I continued. Once again he leaned into me and I knew I had found my way in. The connection had been made.

I worked on him for fifteen to twenty minutes. It was all going very well until suddenly Mike lifted his head and intently looked forward toward the pasture that was only two hundred feet away. There was a string of five mature wolves walking across our line of sight. I had never seen a wolf in the wild, let alone a pack of five. Knowing that the main predator of moose is wolf, I stood next to Mike for several minutes while he watched into the distance not moving a muscle and remaining as still as a statue. I could feel his fear. I could hardly contain my excitement as I realized how much Rolfing SI I had just done while sharing this experience with Mike and the wolves. It felt like he and I had bonded and it was an awesome experience.

Since I could not contain my excitement any longer I rushed into the house to tell Ann about working on Mike and the pack of wolves. Ann was amazed. She had been watching through the window and couldn't believe Mike had been acting so docile. She then told me that ranchers in the area had been having trouble with the wolves occasionally attacking their cattle and because wolves were on the endangered species list it was against the law to shoot them.

It was time for me give Jack a Rolfing session. During the next two hours of my session with Jack, Ann kept giving us updates on Mike's location on their property. As I was doing the session in their living room, I would occasionally take a momentary break to look out the window to see Mike. Frankly, I could hardly wait to complete the session on Jack. At one point Ann reported that Mike was lying down in two feet of snow under a pine tree seventy-five feet away from the house.

When I finished Jack's session I went outside and slowly made my way over to Mike. Mike lay there and made no attempt to get up. I found this fascinating. When I reached him, I knelt down and once again continued the interrupted Rolfing session on him. I started in on his left shoulder

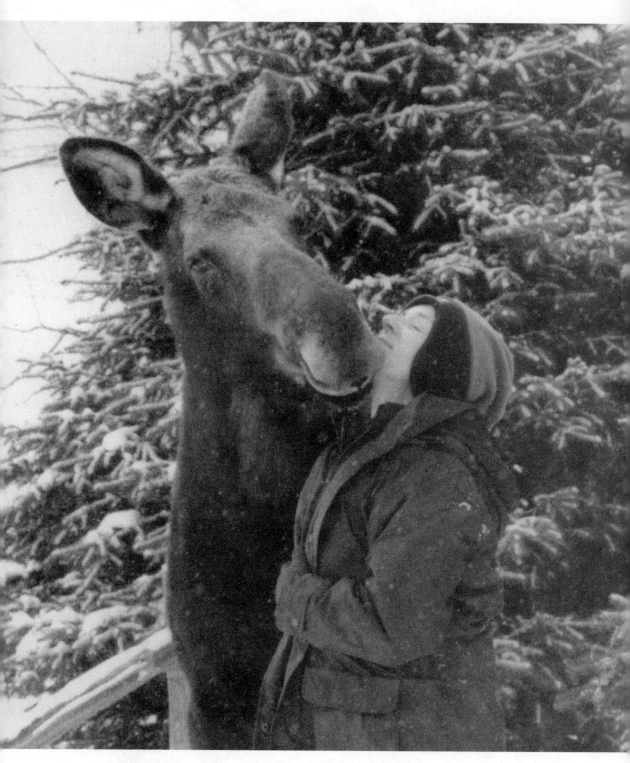

An extraordinary moment. Mike giving me many licks. Photo by Frederick Hirschy.

and gradually worked my way back through the torso. He calmly welcomed the work.

About half an hour into his session, Jack's son, Fred, who was in his forties and owned the adjacent ranch, pulled by in his truck, got out and loudly exclaimed "Oh, that moose hates my guts!" I quietly asked Fred if he would get my camera and take some photos of this experience. As Fred got closer to us, Mike stood up, and so did I, and the strangest thing happened. Mike started licking my entire face with his big long tongue and Fred was able to capture this on film! I have a priceless photo of this. It was the largest tongue that I had ever seen and I was ecstatic with joy. Then Mike did an even more amazing thing—he turned directly around and lay down again, presenting the other side of his back and shoulder to me so I could continue working the other side of him. He knew he needed both sides worked on and wanted to make sure I got the message.

Mike started licking my entire face with his big long tongue. Then Mike did an even more amazing thing—he turned directly around and lay down again, presenting the other side of his back and shoulder to me so I could continue working the other side of him.

I went back into the house as Fred had to leave, and found that Marilyn had finished a Rolfing® session with the cook. I asked her to come outside with me and take more photos. Mike had moved to a different location on the property. He was by a wood fence bordering the yard. I approached Mike, who was standing, and I started to work on him again. As we worked, Mike would stretch his head toward me, into the work, as horses do when I work on them. Marilyn moved closer to take more photos and suddenly Mike felt trapped, with the fence behind him and Marilyn approaching. He put his head down and went after her. Luckily Marilyn was close to the house and escaped in the nick of time. I did not feel any fear for myself as it was clear he was not upset with me, so I continued the session.

As this point he even decided to kneel down, which was amazing not only for the act of submission but it made it easier for me to work on his back. It was as if he knew that this would facilitate his Rolfing session and be much more comfortable. Mind you, Mike stood at least five and a half feet tall, foot to back. I could not have used my elbow to reach his back and torso had he not cooperated by kneeling down in this amazingly intuitive way. It was clear to me that Mike was fully conscious of how this Rolfing session was helping him. So for those people who believe Rolfing SI to be a painful experience, if you could witness these wild animals and their response, you would have an entirely different impression.

It was time for lunch so I suspended my Rolfing session with Mike. I was in the house waiting for Ann to call us to the table. I noticed Mike at a seven-foot high gate outside, standing there and suddenly from a dead stop, I witnessed him leap over that fence. I could not believe his athleticism. I was beginning to have an appreciation for the design of his structure. To me, a moose had seemed to be put together by committee, like a wildebeest. But now I could appreciate how his structure enabled him to be so quick and agile and athletic. I was amazed.

We then left the ranch to go into a nearby town for Ann's doctor visit, other errands and to visit their distant relatives in the valley. This would be our last night in Wisdom at the ranch and I was wondering if I'd see Mike again. Breakfast was in the cookhouse at six o'clock on Sunday, and when we left the main house, lo and behold, we saw Mike standing a mere 100 feet away. He had his ears up as if to eagerly greet us, and about another 150 feet away there was a pair of female moose. He had brought along his harem! After breakfast Mike hung around. I had the opportunity to do a little more Rolfing work. I truly felt as if I'd made a new friend.

I remember calling Ann a week later to check up on Mike. She told me that Mike stayed around the house for three days then disappeared. She thought he was waiting for his Rolfer to come back! I think it was about a month later that I learned that a writer and photographer for *People* magazine had come to Wisdom to do a story about Mike. Mike had appeared and they were able to get a photo of Mike kissing Ann. However, during the photo shoot, Mike managed to kick the photographer. I called back within the next couple of months and they had not seen Mike. As I mentioned in the beginning of the story, it was breeding season and Mike was of mating age. He had other things on his mind.

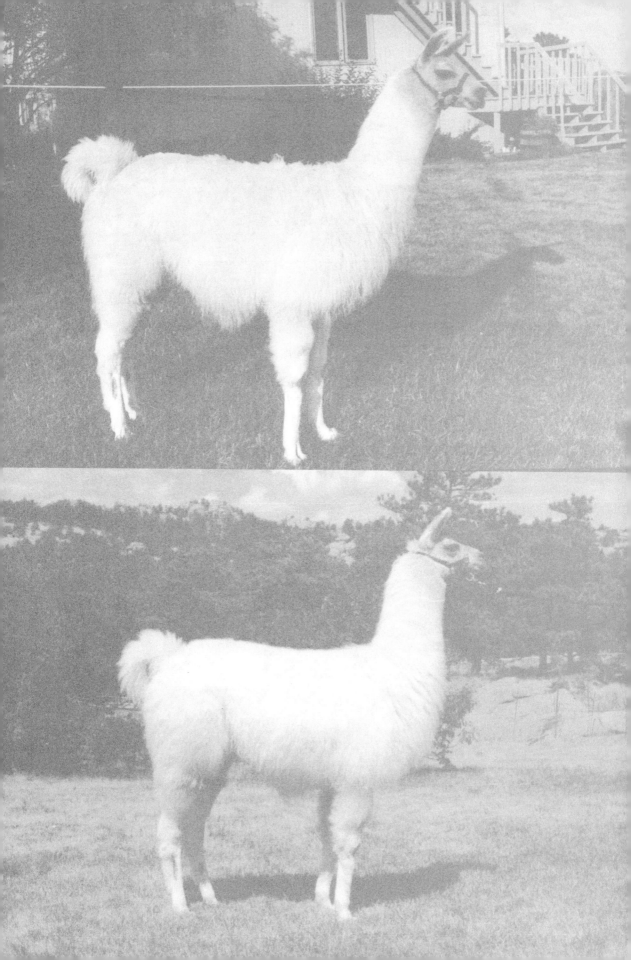

Injury and Rehabilitation

▶ *This is the gospel of Rolfing: when the body gets working appropriately, the force of gravity can flow through. Then, spontaneously, the body heals itself.*

▶ *Rolfing has to do with gravity. Not chemistry, not medicine, not the idea of individually fixing this and that gone wrong. Gravity is the one and only tool that we use. I think my experience justifies making this very broad assumption: gravity is the only tool that deals with chronic situations in the body.*

▶ *Rolfing does not "cure" symptoms. The goal of Rolfing is a more resilient, higher energy system. The organism then is itself better able to defend against illness and overcome stress, and the greater energy does its own beneficial work in healing and relaxing.*

DR. IDA P. ROLF, from *Ida Rolf Talks about Rolfing and Physical Reality*, Rosemary Feitis, ed., Harper Row: NY; 1978

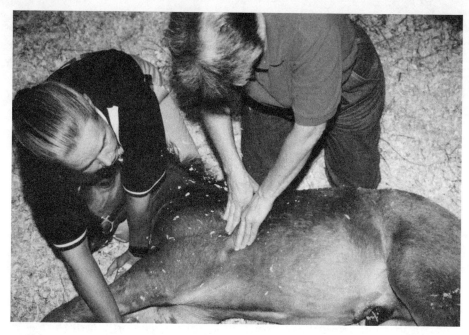

Dr. Julie Wilson assists me as I work with Indy to free and organize his structure.

Rehabilitating Critical Birth Defects

Interview with Dr. Julie Wilson about the foal, Indy

Dr. Julie Wilson is an Associate Professor in the Veterinary Population Medicine department at the University of Minnesota. Her speciality is large animal internal medicine.

Briah Anson: Talk a little bit about how you came to know me and how we collaborated together at the University. I think this was in, was it 2000?

Dr. Julie Wilson: It was a while ago, that's for sure. We had a foal that was donated to the University of Minnesota that was born with a congenital problem due to lack of iodine in the mare's diet while she was pregnant. This baby was born with congenital hypothyroidism and to use the analogy from other species, virtually all mammals need iodine to make thyroid hormones. In frogs, if tadpoles are raised without iodine in their diet, they never go on to mature to be frogs. Horses are somewhat similar in that thyroid hormones, which control metabolism, among other things are critical for normal maturation. So this baby that was donated to the University of Minnesota was born with a number of significant delays in maturation of its body systems.

There are abnormalities that are characteristic of this syndrome leading to a very rapid diagnosis based on just physical examination. The baby's lower jaw is typically longer than the upper jaw, what the horsemen call monkey mouth. Their forelimbs are not able to be fully straightened. They have flexural deformity, and as soon as they try to stand, their lateral digital extensor tends to rupture right where the tendon joins the muscle body. On top of that, the hidden danger is that the small bones that are in the horse's carpals (which would be the equivalent of our wrists), and their hocks (which are like our ankles), are not fully calcified. They are developmentally delayed. So when these babies try to stand up and nurse, which they need to do in the first four hours of life, they begin to crush those bones. That can lead to permanent leg deformity and render them completely useless, and can also lead to very severe arthritis in those joints. We were lucky that we got this baby soon after birth, and it was a great opportunity for our students to see this foal because the clinical signs were so unique; they need to be able to recognize it in the field.

This baby was quite severely affected. There can be a whole range of severity of signs, and this baby was one of the worst ones I have seen. He could not straighten his front legs to a functional level, which meant that he could not get up and try to nurse on his own. He had a lot of tension in his muscle groups associated with those forelimbs that we were unable to address with the tools we had, and that is what led to bringing in Briah to see if she could help us in the process of trying to straighten those limbs by inducing some muscle relaxation with her Rolfing® work.

When Briah came to see Indy, he was three days old, still very young, and the good news was that he had not significantly damaged those small bones in his carpals and hocks so he stood a chance if we could help him

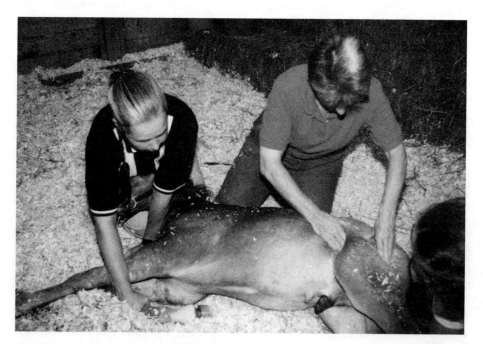

So relaxed he actually went to sleep.

to stand and keep him comfortable. The other issue, too, it is that these babies, if they do stand, need to be supported. They aren't allowed up unless somebody is there with them, and so the additional problem that we frequently have to deal with is that they develop pressure sores from being down all the time. Those

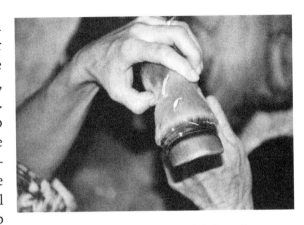

Working intricately to release Indy's front leg.

muscles that are compressed when the baby is down don't have normal circulation either, and you can get into some secondary issues as well.

BA: I recall that I did three sessions on Indy, and they were spaced about a week apart. We would spend one to two hours there working.

JW: In between your visits, we would keep those front legs splinted to protect the carpal bones. It was during that time that the student on the case, Shaun Demmerle, became emotionally bonded with this youngster and he actually ended up officially adopting him because Indy was a donation and would have been euthanized otherwise.

BA: You assisted me in at least in one of the sessions. You had to hold Indy down on the ground. It can be kind of dangerous to hold the foal, the legs can fly.

JW: Imagine a young human child, now gorilla size, who isn't at the stage where they understand what you're saying, and these little legs have tremendous power behind them.

One of the things that most fascinated me with the Rolfing process itself was the foal's reaction. Initially the foal was sort of surprised that people wanted to touch him all over, and yet once Briah began to do her work, he became so relaxed he actually went to sleep, which I thought was fascinating.

The other piece then, is what sort of results did we see? From the veterinarian standpoint that was very significant. Here we were dealing with a young animal that could barely extend his carpal joints past 90 degrees and Briah's help, along with what we were doing with the splints and oxytetracycline therapy to encourage relaxation, really made a difference. When people choose to treat these foals and are willing to put the time and energy into them, I think it's very, very important to recognize that adjunctive therapies like the Rolfing can make a difference. Since that time I have encouraged others that consult with me regarding these hypothyroid foals, to seek out someone willing to work with that baby to encourage muscle relaxation to achieve greater ability to extend those joints, as well as the obvious pleasure that the babies derive from that form of therapy.

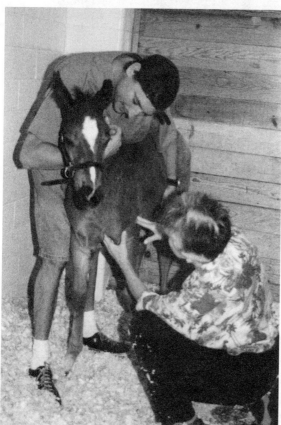

Senior veterinary student, Shaun Demmerle, supports Indy as I work with him standing up.

As part of our routine with this type of baby, we do try to do some extension of the affected joints on a regular basis every time the splints are changed. What we saw was that there was more of a gain in extension than we had seen on the days that the baby did not get a session. The other piece that I thought was really interesting is that gain tended to be sustainable. Sometimes when you do some form of therapy, you see an immediate change but then the next time you assess the animal, you've lost some ground. This was my first experience with Rolfing as an adjunctive therapy and my clinical impression was that the results were more sustainable, and absolutely progressive over the three visits. The results were more sustainable than the usual massage therapy that I had seen on other cases—not congenital hypothyroidism cases, but other horses with musculoskeletal issues.

BA: I remember that by the end of our sessions Indy was walking around quite well and had beautiful conformation.

JW: Right. You know, it took a while to get there, but despite the odds (and most people would have given up on this baby when we first saw him), he did regain the ability to get up and down on his own and to stand with quite straight legs; not perfect, but he did go on to become a functional horse in the pasture. When I spoke some years later with the young man who adopted him, he did say that they ended up doing a releasing surgery to get just a little more gain on that flexural deformity. It has been several years since I spoke with Shaun, but Indy has become a functional, happy horse, although I don't think he is doing anything more than being ridden at a walk.

BA: Any other comments or observations?

JW: What I would really love to see is more application of Rolfing Structural Integration to other cases. I think this foal was an extreme example. There are a lot of foals that have flexural deformities. I would be interested in seeing what sort of progression could be achieved. The therapy that is currently used for some of these is the antibiotic that I mentioned, oxytetracycline, and that comes with some risk. So I think, particularly if we were dealing with a compromised youngster for whom the antibiotic was contraindicated, boy, wouldn't it be nice to be able to get some gains on the extension of those limbs when it is so critical in that early period without having to always resort to splints or oxytetra-cycline. Maybe in the long run we would have better results.

I think there are a lot of applications, and what is exciting about this particular instance is we had a little beast that had been essentially given up on, and we were able to see very visible results, better than anything we expected. I think foals, in particular, are great candidates in which to consider this. Where I don't know if Rolfing would be the appropriate adjunctive therapy is for some of the more acute muscle problems. You know, the sport horses that get tons of muscle injuries and until we try these things I would be speculating.

I think as a profession, as more veterinarians explore adding tools to their toolbox such as acupuncture or chiropractic, there is room to also consider that work on the soft tissues is very, very key. So the trick is going to be putting some objective measures to outcomes to convince

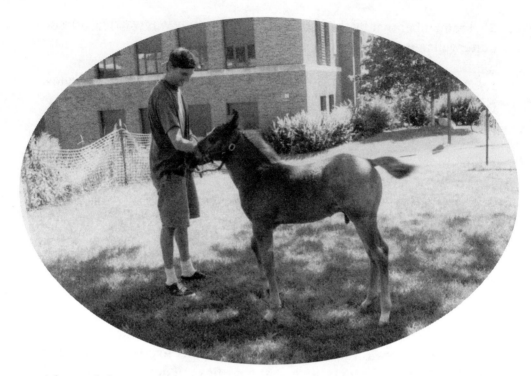

A few weeks later . . . Indy supporting himself, went on to become a functional and happy horse.

the doubters. That would go a long way toward encouraging people to use the modality. For the sport horses that are insured, Rolfing might be covered under their insurance.

My philosophy is that all of our veterinary students should have a broad view of therapies that are potentially available to them as veterinarians, either to learn how to do it themselves or to bring in experts in the field. I was so impressed with the results on Indy that Briah was invited to do a presentation for the veterinary students. This was yet another effort on my part to help them understand ways to integrate therapies into the rehabilitation of patients, and her lecture was very well received and sparked a lot of interest on the students' part.

I would hope that a number of the students that were touched by their interactions with you will then become advocates for this form of therapy and offer that to their clients. I think Rolfing in particular, is not something that horse owners are necessarily aware of. They understand massage and how that has some benefits, but I think the distinction between Rolfing and just any kind of massage is still something that needs more education.

BA: Yes, Rolfing is all connective tissue work that is dealing with a complete restructuring of a horse.

JW: My suspicion is that as more science is applied to this form of therapy in the human field, very similar results will be found when somebody gets around to measuring on the animal side. I hope that happens soon.

Personality and Structure: Integrate and Blossom

Robin Koster and Don Theo Paredes (Peruvian archeologist, anthropologist, and shaman) adopted Tita, a female rottweiler, as a puppy. Robin tells Tita's story.

CUSCO, PERU, 2001. Tita arrived in Poquen Kanchay (Theo's home and healing center) when she was about seven weeks old. She was lankier than Walter, the male Rottweiler that was six months older than she, but seemed like a well-bred dog. She came with papers confirming her full-breed parentage and that her mother did not have hip dysplasia which is congenital in Rottweilers.

On Tita's fifth day with us, we took her on a walk to Tipon, one of the sacred sites nearby. Tipon has terraced walls ranging from three to twelve feet high. I had taken a blanket in case Tita got tired so that I could carry her. But even at such a young age, her desire to keep up with Walter was evident as she wiggled her little body up the stone steps and never stopped running to catch up with him.

Near the end of the day, as we were walking down the terraces to leave, Tita went close to the edge. The grass there was long and gave the illusion that the wall extended further than it did. We tried to pick her up but as she was always a bit apprehensive, our rapid approach caused her to take one step backward. She fell about ten feet. We ran down to her but she was already back up as if nothing had happened. I carried her little wiggling body the rest of the way down. She fought the whole way.

In the days that followed, a few things changed in Tita. The first was that she developed a yeast infection. As it is not unusual for changes to show themselves as imbalances in the body and in females, yeast, I attributed this to her being in a new home and new environment. Then Tita began to cry when we picked her up. We called the vet who came to the house and said that everything was fine. He also said that maybe, even though she had papers saying differently, she was beginning to develop hip dysplasia. He would be unable to determine if this was true until she was six months old, at which time he could take an x-ray.

We feared that this was becoming the reality. As the weeks went by and Tita continued to grow, she never seemed like she was fully in her body. Whereas Walter had grown quickly, one day being fat, the next tall and skinny, then fat, and then tall and skinny, Tita's growth made her look lankier. It seemed as if nothing was sitting right. She continued to be very apprehensive and nervous, which was so different from Walter who was at ease and relaxed. As I had never had puppies before, I could only compare her to Walter and the differences in personality and body form were incredible.

I again talked to the vet who said that Walter had just been a beautiful puppy and told me that there did not seem to be anything wrong with Tita's hips, although we still had some months to wait. Walter and Tita continued to be great friends and they did play very rough. Most thought that it was Walter playing rough but in truth, it was Tita that egged him on. She was growing up to be more aggressive than Walter and I was actually becoming a bit scared. Her apprehension was turning into aggression and walking her in the street became a bit of a challenge. The quick movements of children and their high voices really scared her and she would become aggressive.

I worked a great deal with her, not only trying to break this way of reacting but also trying to encourage her to use her body in different ways. I had heard that one of the best ways to train a dog is to give them as many challenges as possible in their first year. This makes their brain grow and also gives them good body coordination. Tita did okay with the obstacle courses that I would set up but still, I could see that her whole body did not have flexibility. When she moved it was always a bit stiff and awkward. The morning stretches were also a clue. Walter would stretch his front legs completely out in front of him and then do the same with his back legs. Tita never stretched out her back legs.

All of this left me feeling very sad at the thought that when she became six months old, an X-ray would reveal that she had hip dysplasia and the kindest thing to do, I had heard, was put the dog to sleep. As we were in Peru, there was no option of surgery.

When Briah arrived and told me that she was a Rolfer™ who worked on animals and offered to work on Walter, I almost cried. I began to tell her about Tita and all of the observations that I had made. She told me that she would work on Tita when she arrived at Poquen Kanchay in a few days.

Briah did three very long deep sessions with Tita. The photos of these sessions show a lot of apprehension in Tita's eyes. They also show her stance—like a scared cat. I was not here during the sessions but the before and after differences I could see in the photos were very apparent.

The first thing that I noticed upon my return was Tita's walk. For the first time, she looked as if she was in her body. She seemed much more grounded and at home, and consequently moved with agility and ease. I took a picture of Tita barking one week after the sessions with Briah. The difference in her little body is incredible. She was very alert in the photo so her whole body was tense, but she looked very at ease and beautiful and her muscles well-defined in a way I hadn't seen before. It was as if after four months of being held by strings, something had let go and everything fell into place. Her bones, her muscles, her skin—it all fit.

Then there were our daily walks. As we live in the country, the walks always included jumping over water or logs, up little hills and down. This new Tita was like a little antelope, jumping off the ground with all four paws at the same time, as if she had springs in her feet. I had never seen

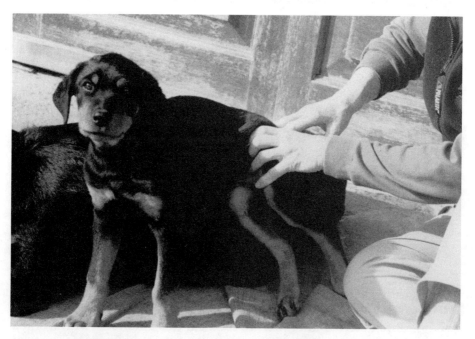

Tita, a three-month-old rottweiler receiving her first session. I'm working here on her twisted hind end.

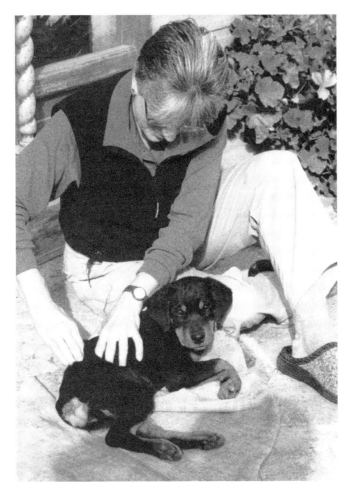

Later in the session; Tita relaxing and feeling comfortable with my touch.

anything like it. And she was happy, much more confident, not always hiding by my side. In character and body, she was a very different dog.

She is still very different from Walter, not as trusting as he is and always more alert. She is also still very competitive with him and when they play, they both share equally in the fight. But she is so much happier than she was before, and much more at ease. We have had no problems with her barking or growling at children and she does not try to pick fights with other dogs. And this jumping thing has never stopped—every morning when I pick up her food bowl, she jumps into the air. It is her way to show how happy she is to be alive! It's a movement that is filled with excitement and joy.

We did have her X-rayed and there is no problem with her hips. Briah had told us that even if she had a genetic tendency to hip displasia, it probably wouldn't show up as a movement problem after the Rolfing. I attribute what happened to Tita to be caused by her fall and not genetic. It was not until a few months after Briah was here that I remembered the fall.

After Tita's first heat, her body changed a lot in only a two-week period. But again, I thanked Briah—it seemed to me that the changes happened without resistance and Tita moved through her heat with a flexible body that allowed for growth in some areas and then after the heat, the reduction again. She has now stopped growing, and she is a very fine Rottweiler, toned, trim, agile, muscular, alert, and very loving.

I will always look at Briah's coming as a gift sent by angels, as I love my dogs very much! I thank her with all my heart because she helped Tita not only in body but also in spirit.

Mary Rutherford is a chiropractor from St. Paul, Minnesota, who leads shamanic trips to Peru. Here she relates her observations of Tita and experiences with Rolfing SI.

In April of 2000, my daughter Morgan and I, together with Briah, were on a trip down to Peru. Robin, who worked in Theo's office at the time, had asked me before we came if Briah would be willing to do some Rolfing sessions on Tita. She told me that they had done a lot of research on her breeding and thought that she had hip dysplasia. She didn't remember until after Briah had worked on her that she had fallen off of a fourteen-foot wall at Tipon. They actually thought they might have to have her put down if she developed a painful arthritis.

Upon our arrival we met Tita and Walter. Walter was already an adult and Tita was just a puppy that they had adopted to breed with him. At times you see dogs that walk as if their back legs aren't behind their front legs, they're kind of off to the side, and that's how Tita looked to me. My eye isn't trained to look at the structure of a dog, but I could see that she was catawampus.

Briah did a couple of sessions with Tita at Theo's house where we were staying. Since then, I have seen her many times because I usually go there once or twice a year. Theo was thrilled that Tita did not develop hip dysplasia and have to be put down. In fact, she never developed any problems at all and she just grew into a normal dog after that major fall.

It is now November, 2009, and Tita is nine years old. When I was there in June I took some pictures of her, and she is gorgeous. She looks young and very regal in her stature. She has a little bit of gray hair but other than that she looks very youthful. She's active, she runs around and jumps. She doesn't have any problems at all. This is a totally different outcome from the direction she seemed to be going when she was young. She's well behaved but she's happy and runs around freely. No hip issues at all. She has had at least two litters that I know of, so she was successful in that. Her puppies were very healthy.

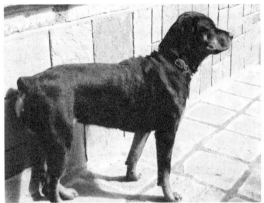

Tita nine years later! She has developed into a strong, self assured, and beautifully aligned dog. Photos by Mary Rutherford.

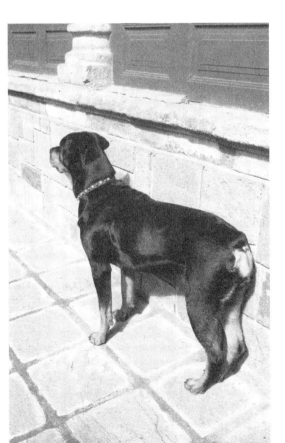

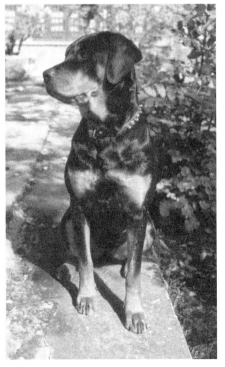

Tita had been really shy and not as outgoing as Walter, but after she had the Rolfing sessions she just blossomed. She is really comfortable with people now. As soon as I walk in the gate, she runs up wiggling and wants to be petted. She loves people. I didn't detect any shyness even from the first day that I showed up, and I hadn't seen her in a year. I don't assume she remembers me since there are so many people that come there, and she's really comfortable with people coming in.

I know that Rottweilers have a reputation for being aggressive and that some people take advantage of that and train them to be that way, but what I observed in Tita after Rolfing is that she is neither aggressive nor shy. She seems very well socialized. She enjoys people a lot. I have never seen her jump up on anybody or run away from them. It is really healthy behavior in every way. She is very comfortable and confident with herself. She doesn't shy away from people or situations, and there are a lot of different people who come in there—little kids, big men, loud people, quiet—she seems comfortable with all those different situations.

Around the same time that Tita was Rolfed, my daughter Morgan had just completed her Rolfing series with Briah. Morgan was twelve years old at the time, and I saw similar changes happen in her. I had taken her to a different Rolfer at first and didn't see anything change and was a little frustrated with that. After four sessions, nothing, and I have enough of an eye for structure to see that nothing was happening. I asked the other Rolfer why nothing was changing, and she said, "She's not ready." So I thought, well, what I need is a different Rolfer, not a different daughter!

So I brought her to Briah, who did the 10-series on her (which the other woman had not done) and she just blossomed. So I knew to watch for a similar kind of change in Tita.

What I have observed about Briah's work is that her gift is unique from the ten Rolfers I've been to over the years, in that she is able to see the future. I don't know what that is about or how she does it. Nobody else that I've been to does that. She sees the future potential in the structure and brings it out. I don't know if she intends that, or is thinking about that when she's working, but that's exactly what I see her do. The kids that Briah works on grow up beautifully.

To bring this back to Tita's story: Briah Rolfed her when she was little, and she became who she came on earth to be. Just like Tita before Rolfing, Morgan used to be extremely shy. It was a challenge to get her to speak in certain situations. People would ask her questions and she wouldn't answer. I found myself answering for her at times because she just didn't say anything. Sometimes I regret that I did that because it didn't help her find her own voice, but she just didn't say anything. She was extremely shy and I think Rolfing and homeopathy were the two things that brought her forth. One of the homeopaths that I brought her to when she was six years old handed me her remedy and said, "Now she can be who she came on earth to be." That's what happened with Tita as well.

I think people, animals, and even plants, have an agenda they're born with. We came here to do a certain thing and to be a certain thing. Plants have decided that they're not going to move for their entire life, that they're going to just be planted, so to speak; animals move around so we need a different kind of structure to move around with, but we still have that agenda for our entire lives. Sometimes things get in the way and we can't fully become what we had intended. I know it's a big mystery.

Morgan is now twenty-three. She is in design school, working toward her masters in architecture. When she gives presentations in front of committees now, she's totally confident. She stands up there, very striking looking because her structure is very grounded and upright. She had twelve years of education before college that led her to develop this interest in art and gave her a skill at speaking in front of groups of people. She has big goals. She wants to focus on designing hospitals and clinics. She has visions for the way that hospital rooms should be designed for healing, and I am so glad that somebody is finally going to do that!

Morgan is now a very confident young woman, and that comes through in her voice even on the telephone. Her brain is wired so that she can express herself clearly, and now that she has lost the shyness, she can say what she thinks. She doesn't have the inner angst that a lot of people develop from all the stresses of life. She has continued to go to a homeopath and to get her structure straightened around.

In observing both Morgan and Tita over the years, I have seen them develop balanced structures and balanced personalities. They're integrated. I guess that's where the term Structural Integration comes from! The whole personality and the structure integrate so that there's a groundedness and clarity. Morgan's thinking and Tita's behavior reflect how they feel on the inside.

Acute Spinal Injury and the Treatment that Worked

Asea Cole, on her greyhound, Coco

We adopted Coco shortly after the loss of our other adopted greyhound. His racing name was Yukon Cornelius, and the adoption agency had named him "Corn." For Coco and me, it was love at first sight! I had visited a much younger greyhound, but the chemistry just wasn't there. I decided to visit "Corn," who had just been neutered and had a bunch of teeth pulled out. He was six years old. When "Corn" was let in the room, he came toward me, tail wagging, and gave me a big kiss . . . it was as if he was saying, "Where have you been? I've been waiting for you!"

"Corn" was a racing greyhound. When the racetracks in Hudson closed, his racing owner kenneled him in his house. Unfortunately, he was not well cared for. When we adopted "Corn," he was being treated for parasites and had had many teeth pulled out, including all of his front bottom teeth and a canine.

"I can't have a dog named Corn!" I said. "How about Corn Dog?" my husband replied. "We can call him Popcorn!" exclaimed my son. "Coco," I said, for Corn Cole (our last name).

Since Coco had been kenneled most of his life, it took him about ten days to feel safe enough to get out of the kennel and hang out with the rest of the family. To our delight, he was self-entertaining—he would play fetch by himself, tossing his stuffed animals (or those of my daughter) and run and pounce after it. None of our other adopted greyhounds had ever played like that so Coco's playing was fun for us to watch. He was also the fastest greyhound we had ever adopted. He ran like the wind! Life was good at the Cole residence once again.

Then one cold January day when I was home alone with Coco, I let him out in the fenced yard to do his business. Soon I heard a loud animal cry. When I looked outside, Coco was on his rear, spinning around in a circle. I went outside and lifted his back side, but his paws were curled inward and he would not, could not, stand on his feet. I knew something was wrong. I called my neighbors and found someone who could help me carry him from the backyard to my car. In the meantime I had called and found an emergency vet who could take him in.

The diagnosis was not good. They said he was paralyzed. He had most likely ruptured a disc and we could either take him to the University vet hospital for back surgery, or put him to sleep right away or . . . wait and see! I opted to wait and see. They kept him in the emergency clinic and managed his pain until the next day when I transported him back to our regular vet. They continued pain management medications but encouraged me to stop his pain and suffering if we did not want to go ahead with an expensive back surgery. I remember thinking that this wasn't fair. Coco had just started having a good life. It could not end so soon!

In the meantime, I had called a chiropractor friend of the family, Dr. Reza, for help. I knew he owns and loves horses and dogs and asked him if there was anything he could do for Coco. He agreed to come to our vet's office (a very long drive away) and check him out. He gave Coco a spinal treatment and encouraged us to give him time to heal. Based on his recommendation, we moved Coco to the University of Minnesota intensive care unit for pain management.

Coco seemed to be making some progress under the vet's care. I would go and visit Coco every day for about an hour. They used to bring him from ICU in a red wagon to the visiting area and lay him down on towels and I would lay down next to him and rub his back and neck, telling him how much I loved him and that he had to get better. He had just begun to finally have a good life . . . I could not let it end so quickly. I would not!

In the meantime, I found a vet who specializes in greyhounds, Dr. Barr. He gave us the encouraging news that the majority of greyhounds can recover from this kind of trauma, but he had to examine Coco to determine his chances. So I transported Coco from the University to Foley Animal Hospital in Coon Rapids.

It was there that for the first time I had any hopes of recovery for Coco. The attending technician shared the story of her greyhound who was older than Coco, and was now able to get around fairly well after a few months of nursing and caring. The vet warned us that greyhounds recover more quickly in a home environment. So there I was with a seventy-plus pound paralyzed greyhound! He needed to be carried up the stairs, kept in a diaper, and flipped from side-to-side every two hours to avoid bed sores and further complications!

The home care was tough! I slept on the sofa in the living room at night so I could be near Coco whose bed we had now moved to the kitchen. Every couple of hours I would get up, change his diaper and bed pads and move him from side to side. In the morning, I would take him back to the vet for observation while I worked and would pick him up after work.

Fortunately, Coco started showing slow signs of improvement. Soon, I could stand him up and help him empty his bladder. Then he got to the point where he could stand, but we could see how crooked his spine was; it looked like a question mark!

Once Coco could stand on his own and walk very slowly, dragging his left leg, I made an appointment with Briah for my annual Rolfing® treatments and mentioned Coco's story to Briah. She suggested I take him along on my next appointment.

Coco could barely walk to Briah's office and needed my help up the stairs. But Briah soon made him comfortable in her office and started working on him. The expression on Coco's face was priceless! Briah worked on Coco for an hour and then he rested there as Briah worked

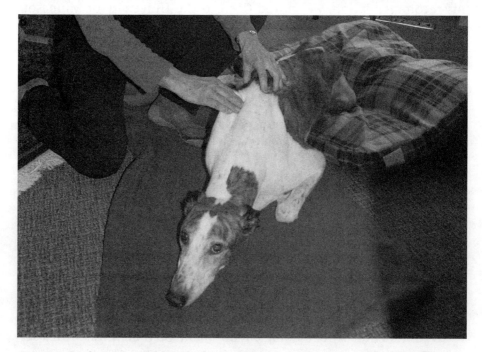

Coco, a retired racing greyhound who could barely walk into my office, being comforted and healed.

her miracle on my body (that is another unbelievable miracle story all by itself). When it was time to leave, Coco was reluctant and needed a lot of pulling and tugging on his leash to be taken away from Briah's office. Was it his animal sense telling him that she was there to help him? As I was taking him to the car, I noticed the "question mark" spine looked straight! But I kept it to myself. When we got home, the kids noticed how straight his spine was, too.

Briah worked on Coco two more times. It was the same story each time: Coco excited about going to the office, and reluctant about leaving Briah! He loved being Rolfed and then rested comfortably as Briah worked on my body.

As I tell this story, it has been seven months since Coco's mishap when he ruptured a disc in his spine. The "miracle boy," as I call him, is now walking on his own and is looking for any opportunity to run, even though he is not supposed to!

After the miracle Briah had made in my own life (I was suffering from chronic pain of fibromyalgia until Briah Rolfed me), I was not surprised at all about the changes she made in Coco's life. Coco has had an amazing recovery and continues a happy life as a "retired" racing greyhound. . . . Much thanks to Briah and her Rolfing.

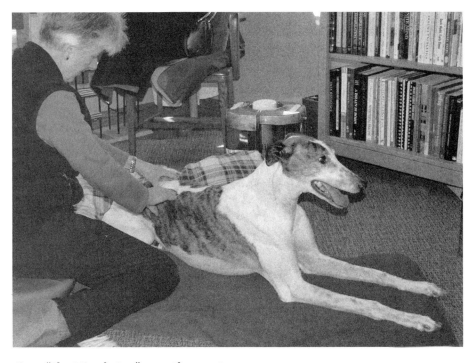

Coco, "The Miracle Boy" . . . on the way to recovery.

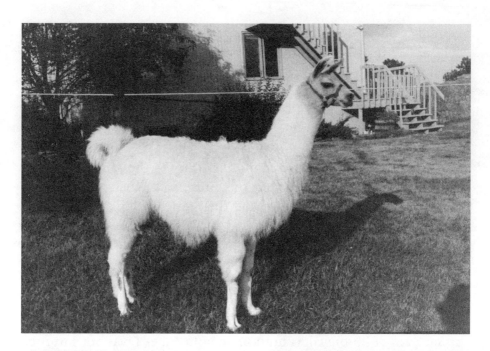

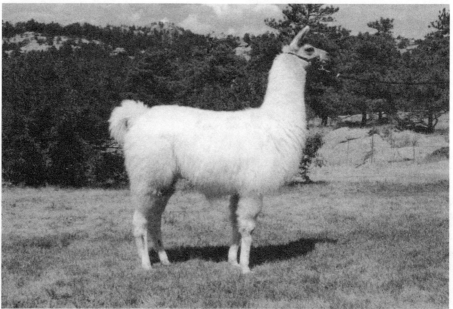

Top. *Larry before Rolfing® SI: showing some misalignments and shortness through his body. Note how his pelvis is torqued, his legs don't support him in an optimal position and his head is not as upright as it could be.* **Bottom.** *Larry after 2 sessions: More upright and squarely aligned, his legs giving him support and now showing a beautiful conformation.*

The Llamas of Boulder Ridge Ranch

Briah recalls her first experience working with llamas

In the summer of 1993 I traveled to Estes Park, Colorado, to attend the Rolf Institute® annual meeting. While in Colorado I took the opportunity to work with some llamas I had been invited to visit. One of my clients had a sister and brother-in-law who own a llama ranch in Lyons, Colorado, and I was interested in the possibility of working with llamas. I was invited to stay at Bob and Jo Reilly's home for a couple of days and it was there that I would work on three of their llamas.

The first was a young llama by the name of Larry who was very sweet and docile, and was a wonderful introduction for me in how to work with a llama and discover their nature. I then worked with Areesh, a large black and white male who was a bit more challenging because of his size and his attitude, but that gave me more confidence. At the end of the day as I was leaving, I noticed that in their pasture there was a young, white, very small llama and pointed it out to them. It was a llama that had been born just a few hours earlier. I had another hour before I needed to leave, so I did a session on this young llama who they later decided to name Briah, after myself.

Bob and Jo shared with me that they had a friend who had a large male llama, Chief, that was used for breeding that had been seriously injured, and they were wondering if I might be able to give this llama a Rolfing® session. I was heading off to the meeting in Estes Park, but I agreed that on the return from my conference I could spend one more day at their house and see what I could do regarding this big black male.

Camacho Chief is Introduced to Rolfing SI

When Alaine Byers purchased Camacho Chief Indian Peaks from Dick Patterson, Chief was five months old—a large black woolly llama standing tall and straight as an arrow, destined to be Alaine's herd shire at Indian Peaks Ranch in Ward, Colorado. Alaine was so proud of him that she took him to the International Llama and Alpaca conference in Salt Lake City. Alaine was not going straight home after the conference so a fellow Colorado breeder offered to transport him back along with some of his llamas. It was immediately apparent something had happened to Chief. He went down and would not rise. At Colorado State University he was diagnosed as having suffered trauma to the sacral region. A breeder with a good eye commented that he was "camped under," an appearance suggesting a genetic defect.

When the body is injured, i.e., a sprained ankle, bruised calf muscle or a herniated disk, as might have been the case with Chief, the body will repair itself by pulling muscles in a way to support the injured area and relieve the pain. However, the fascia or sheath surrounding the muscle tissue does not return to its original position. Human beings accumulate little bumps and bruises and over time our bodies get out of balance and we develop "poor conformation" as had happened to Chief. Chief was now five years old and still camped under. I had done Rolfing sessions not only on people but also many animals, both wild and domestic, so agreed to work with Chief.

Chief was born in July of 1988 and about a year later he developed what they thought was colic the day after returning from the trip to the International Llama and Alpaca conference in Salt Lake City. They took him to Colorado State University where they did a whole series of exams including a belly tap and blood workups, and concluded that he had had some kind of traumatic injury to his lower back—his sacral area, which had affected his stance and his gait.

Pre-session Observations
After hearing this story from Alaine about Chief's history, I did a gait analysis of Chief's walk. His gait was way off. His rear legs didn't track straight ahead, and neither did his front legs; it seemed that his right rear leg crossed the midline. Alaine commented that his gait was very stiff and jerky, and that she often wondered if that indicated that he was in pain. She reported that trying to get Chief to square off or move in a smooth

motion was almost impossible. When Chief stopped walking he placed his feet in the positions that would accommodate his compensations.

I explained to Alaine that with the Rolfing process, the purpose would be to align Chief's body in the field of gravity, to systematically organize the segments of his body in such a way that there would be symmetry and balance and have each of the segments working appropriately. This would then translate into good functional movement. I explained to Alaine that I wanted to free up his shoulder girdle and his breathing first, and then organize the front legs as they connect up into the shoulder. I would then lengthen his torso on both sides and free up his spine, and then proceed to focus on freeing up the pelvic area. This would include creating more space in the lumbosacral area, freeing his entire pelvis and organizing the rear legs into his pelvis.

No vet and not even the Colorado State University had been able to do anything for him. Was it possible to rectify the health of this being, relieve his suffering and give him a new lease on life?

Since I only had one day at their ranch, I set out to do what typically would have been a three-to-four-session process, with sessions lasting an hour and a half to two hours each. I worked about two-thirds of the day with an hour break. The reason for this was because Chief had been in such an acute condition for so long and no one, no vet and not even the team at Colorado State University had been able to do anything for him, so this was clearly an experiment to see what was possible. Was it possible to rectify the health of this being, relieve his suffering and give him a new lease on life?

I noticed that there was a significant amount of compression at his head to neck juncture and that the carriage of his neck was not as vertical as it could be. I noticed that Chief did not exhibit much freedom of movement in his body. Each of his body movements seemed to move in a restricted way and there was very little fluidity to his overall movement patterns. He was unable to hold his tail up in a centrally located position as a llama with good movement patterns would.

The Sessions

When I first approached Chief, he pulled away from me. It was obvious that he did not want to be touched. I gently continued to talk to him and approach him, but could not even get within two feet without him yanking hard on the lead rope. Alaine mentioned that they had not been able to do anything with him, i.e., brush him, or do anything unless they put him in a chute. We put him in a chute where his neck and head were restrained by bars on either side so that he could not turn or spit on me (this spit is hurled with great speed and force and can be painful and unpleasant to receive).

There was a wooden gate that came up about three feet on either side so Chief would not be able to kick his handlers. I then proceeded to start working on his left shoulder area. He immediately started to spit and kick a bit. Alaine had tried to do massage and the Tellington Touch technique on him, and she had had this same angry reaction from him. Almost immediately as I started to work with Chief, he responded by shifting the weight of his legs back and forth as he attempted to find a new balance point.

Within a few minutes Chief started to settle and made sounds that signaled more acceptance of the work. He was no longer grunting, spitting and yanking his neck and head in the chute. As I worked the ring around his pelvic region, I observed him working with me to find better foot placement with his rear legs. He would actually lean his left rear side into me as I worked in that area. Alaine noted that his eyes had softened and looked glazed over. His ears were forward and his breathing was deeper and more relaxed.

After about an hour of work we took Chief out of the chute so that we could observe how these structural changes were translating into new movement patterns. What we observed was that his front legs were tracking in a straight ahead direction and we observed that his rear legs were under his pelvis and tracking better without crossing the midline. His overall structure was looking much freer and he was moving with fewer restrictions.

We then went back to the chute for the next session and as I started to work on his back, close to his thoracic lumbar area, I shared with Alaine my experience of doing Rolfing sessions on a cougar a few years earlier. I told her about the cougar being quite aggressive during the initial part of his first session, and how, after about half an hour of this struggle, the cougar finally lay down and was so relaxed that I was able to have one of my dreams come true, which was being able to lay on the cougar. It was at this moment that Chief immediately lay down in the chute. Whether this was a coincidence or not, it was a remarkable moment for both Alaine and I as it seemed to us that Chief was listening and tracking this story. We felt he was saying, "if it's good enough for a cougar, it's good enough for me."

I then knelt down and started working the tissues in a much deeper way. I was moving many layers of stuck tissue and could feel the tissues being built up and feeling softer and more resilient. At this point, Chief was laying his head down on the ground and his eyes were almost closed. His ears were relaxed and he was breathing in a deeper rhythm. I proceeded to work at the juncture of his head and neck and he remained calm and still.

Results

After this productive period of work, I felt that we'd reached the conclusion of this session of work. We took him out of the chute to observe him walking. Tim, his handler, walked Chief and then brought him to a halt, and Chief squared off perfectly. Alaine had never seen Chief be able to do that and this was done without any coaching on the part of the handler. As we watched him walk, we noticed how he picked up his front legs effortlessly and how his rear legs tracked straight ahead like a well oiled machine. There were no hitches in his pelvis and his hind end looked fuller and

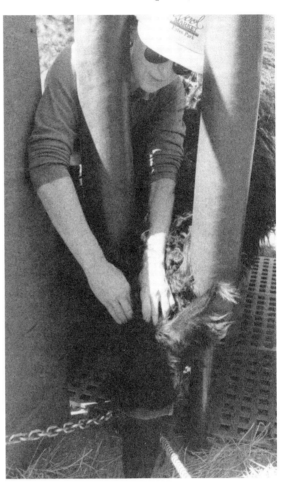

Working on Chief in a holding chute!

higher. As a matter of fact, his entire structure looked several sizes fuller. Alaine remarked that he no longer looked round-rumped and dumpy. He did not look so earthbound. His head was not as far forward and he had much more vertical lift with his neck and head.

At the completion of this day of concentrated Rolfing sessions, Alaine walked with Chief and said, "I hardly had to move him to place him. It's really amazing. He just looks square. Even if he does not put his left back leg forward, he still lines up square because his back end is squared." She went on to say that she would expect that as the days go on, Chief will

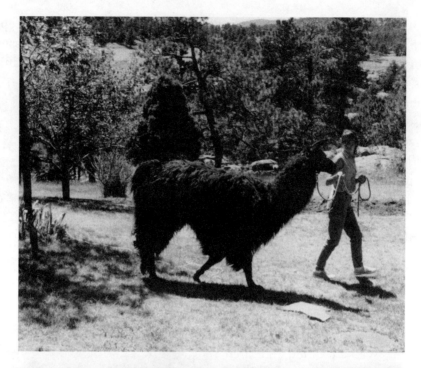

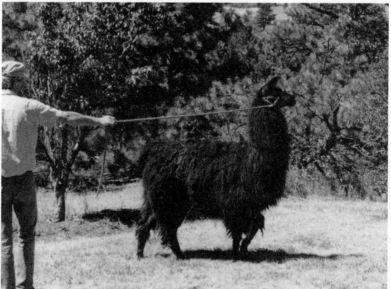

Top. *Chief walking before any Rolfing® work in a difficult and lumbering manner.* **Bottom.** *After several sessions in one day: Chief looking well organized, proud, upright, and moving with grace and elegance.*

feel more accustomed to feeling like this and holding himself up like he is today.

One of the prinicples of Rolfing SI is that as you change the major segments of the body to line up to do what they are intended to do, you can then get the body working and moving appropriately with grace and ease.

When Alaine and Chief returned home, she couldn't believe how he acted. He ran into the field and jumped around. He now breeds for forty-five minutes instead of his previous fifteen-minute breedings. Getting Chief ready for a show had always been hard. When Alaine would put her hand on Chief's back, he would spit at her. Now she can touch him anywhere without a reaction. Alaine says that Chief is "a totally different llama" as a result of this Rolfing series. Alaine later reported that nine months after the Rolfing experience, all the improvements in Chief had remained. The most wonderful part of the whole experience, Alaine reported, is to see an animal that had been in pain for years be suddenly relieved of that pain. Although Chief could have used additional Rolfing work, Alaine was so confident in his progress that she planned on showing him at the ALSA llama show in Estes Park that next year.

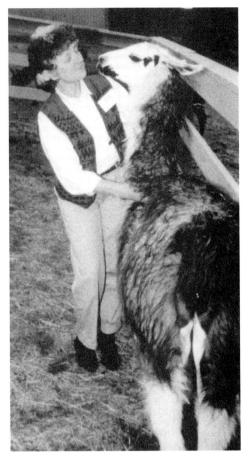

I gave Briah (my namesake) a Rolfing® SI session when she was only hours old. This reunion occurred a year later. I watched her run in the pasture and she had the most beautiful and free gait I had seen in a llama.

As a result of this experience, I was invited the following summer to attend the International Llama and Alpaca conference in Boulder, Colorado. I was given a two-hour time slot where I could present the theoretical basis of Rolfing Structural Integration, show many slides of my work with animals and people, and give my experience of working with Chief. This was a remarkable experience for me because it was the first introduction of Rolfing SI to the llama and alpaca community.

As Good As New: Healing after Back Injury

Abbey Hutson, on her dog, Herschell

Hershell is a rescue dog, and as far as we know he is part bassett and part beagle, about ten years old now. He is a short dog with a very long back and he weighs about forty pounds. When I brought Herschell in to be Rolfed in January of 2007 he was just about seven years old.

Herschell sustained a bad back injury when a woman grabbed him and picked him up improperly. He has a very long back and this woman grabbed him quickly under his front two legs so his back was hanging down in the air and the back half of his body was unsupported. He cried out and I ran over as quickly as I could to support the lower half of his body but the injury had already happened. Over the following few days he kept getting worse and worse. One January day I was out walking Herschell and, this being Minnesota, there was a lot of snow. He had gone over a pile of snow to sniff, and when he tried to jump back over the pile, his two back legs went out behind him. He shrieked in pain and he couldn't move, so I had to carry him part of the way back home.

I had already been looking for things to do to help his back injury and had been treating him homeopathically with Hypericum and another remedy, but there was not much effect from the remedies. So my homeopath told me to go see Briah and get Herschell some Rolfing® work. It was amazing. He only had two Rolfing sessions for this injury, and after the very first session he was 95 percent back to normal, maybe even 100 percent. He didn't have any more episodes of pain after the first Rolfing session and he didn't have any more trouble moving or walking.

When I brought him to that first session, he relaxed into it right away and he just seemed to know that it was helping him. He lay on the floor while Briah Rolfed him. It lasted almost an hour and then when he was ready and felt finished, he just got up and walked off. He was able to walk normally after that session, whereas before he was having such problems with it. He hasn't had an episode of pain since the first Rolfing session but Briah wanted me to bring him back for a second session. I think it was really helpful as it solidified what had happened in the first session.

I think the second Rolfing session was about two or three weeks after the first one. In that second session, Briah worked more with his pelvis which was where the main injury occurred. Herschell's always been a really happy dog and after the Rolfing he was able to get back to his normal self. He's a sweetheart. Since those first sessions I've brought him back for a session or two every year.

I'm trained as a homeopath, and I have to say I don't understand a lot about Rolfing, but I do know from my experience with Herschell it was the only thing that was able to support him in a way that allowed him to heal from his injury. The homeopathic remedies were not able to do that. Remedies are amazing; they can do a lot of things, but for a physical injury like he had, the Rolfing was what he needed.

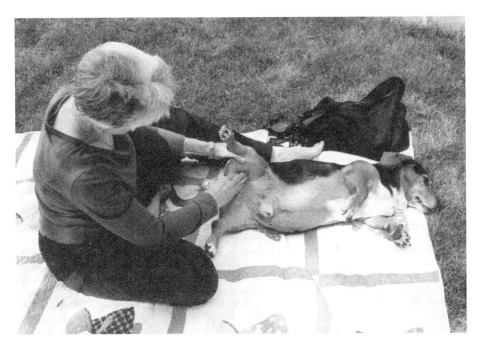

Herschell, a bassett/beagle mix, cooperating beautifully as I work in a vulnerable area of his pelvis.

I'm going to keep getting Herschell Rolfing sessions because I believe that it's helpful to his overall support. I try to do lots of things to help him live as long and as well as he can. This Rolfing work is a really important piece of what I provide for him, especially since he is a dog with a long, vulnerable back, and a little low to the ground. I think it can be beneficial for all dogs, but especially for the ones who are prone to hip or back problems.

I exercise Herschell as much as I can. I take him on long walks which he has no trouble with. He has had other health problems, like low blood sugar, that I have been able to treat homeopathically. The Rolfing has been beneficial for his overall health and injury repair, and I think he's less vulnerable to injuries now because his structure is more in alignment.

Now at age ten, Herschell acts exactly like he did at age five. He's very happy and he's very agile. He has a lot of energy. He gets excited at the appropriate times and he's mellow at the appropriate times. He likes to go for long walks. He likes to get out and sniff in the woods and chase rabbits when he can. I think he has quite a few healthy years left, and I attribute that to the Rolfing, homeopathy, and good supportive care of his homeopathic veterinarian.

I'm so grateful to Briah for working with animals because this has been such a blessing in my life. If Herschell hadn't been Rolfed things could have turned out very differently because it was a really serious injury. Rolfing can completely change the direction of a pet's trajectory. It's amazing and simple.

Injury—The Gateway to Confidence

Anne Schuerger, on her dog, Clancy

Clancy is a two-year-old golden retriever. He was a tiny pup when we got him and it appeared to me from the start that he was a bit timid and not terribly coordinated. I remember the first time that we saw him on the back porch of the woman's house where he lived. It was slippery with wet leaves and he, of all the pups, was the one that was falling down, slipping around and sliding the most. He was just delightful. As we did the temperament testing and checking in with the different dogs and how we felt about them, he seemed to be the one for us. He wasn't the runt of the litter; he definitely appeared a little smaller and a little less coordinated than the other dogs, but he had the temperament that we wanted.

Clancy's Injury

He grew normally, but he was never the kind of the dog that ran with abandon. He would play and be joyful but mostly he would roll—he loved to roll and put his legs in the air. Clancy would run, but never full out, and could not sustain running for very long. He was almost always subservient with other dogs and people. Clancy was a little over a year old when I started the Rolfing® series for myself, and I wondered if there was something Rolfing might do to help him organize his movement a bit more.

When he was a little less than a year old a major incident occurred. It had been raining and the grass was wet. The neighbor dog, who was significantly smaller than Clancy, was over to play. For some reason Clancy slipped and when he stood up he was holding his left hind leg up. I knew immediately that he was in a lot of pain. He held it out stiffly for a while hobbling around on three legs and looking quite taken aback. He lay down and I immediately applied ice to keep the swelling down.

It improved over the next couple of days but I eventually took him to a vet. The first vet we saw watched him walk but didn't do a technical examination because Clancy was protecting his leg and wouldn't let the vet close to it. The vet said, "Oh, he has torn his ACL and he is going to need surgery," and explained what would be involved. My husband and I researched the surgery, looked Clancy over, and said, "Hmm, I'm not so sure."

We got a second and a third opinion. The vet who gave us a second opinion said, "Well, I'm not sure." The third vet did the actual technical testing for movement in the joint. He was testing for lateral movement that would indicate whether the tendons and soft tissues were really gone, broken or out of whack. Clancy wasn't very happy about it. The vet said, "I'm not so sure. You could very well do this surgery and still find that he is not getting full range of motion or he is not fully weight-bearing on it." So we just decided it was way too big a surgery for this young a pup without knowing if it was really an issue. That was just about the time that I started Rolfing and it occurred to me to say "Hey, Briah, I see that Golden Retriever on your wall," and we got to talking about it, and it just made sense to bring him in to see what she could do with him.

Clancy had three Rolfing sessions. The first two were about two weeks apart and the third was a month later. In the first session, it was very new to him being touched in that way, and he clearly enjoyed it. He was just over a year at that point so he was still a little bit squirrelly in his ability to relax in a new space. I remember that we did it in rounds—about ten minutes of really concentrated relaxation where he was experiencing the Rolfing and going into that internal state, and then he would get squirrelly and Briah would just let him be. At one point he actually presented the other side to Briah which I thought was really interesting. I brush him constantly because he is a therapy dog and has to be clean, but he rarely understands when I want him to turn on the other side. Even after all those months of brushing, he will rarely let me turn him around. But this looked like he was saying, "Oh, that felt good, now could you do the other side?" I think Briah started with the uninjured side first, and then he offered the other side which was definitely different. He didn't do his usual protecting on that side while Briah was working on him.

The first session lasted about an hour, opening up his breathing, working his whole shoulder girdle, working down the spine and a little bit of work on the hind end. I had the sense afterward that there had been something kind of crooked about him, and he now seemed a little more square. His legs had been splayed out and now they were more underneath him. He looked more vertical, like his legs were bearing downward instead of out through the hip sockets, especially in the back end. Briah was primarily working on the front end, but he organized through the whole body.

We go to the dog park just about every day and after the second session we noticed that he was more able to really dig in when he was running. We started going to a dog park that has a sandy area of forest and he would take off running in big circles around us, just really digging in. It looked like he was beginning to get his back to arch so that when he was running, those rear legs would come underneath him and push off. I had never seen him run like that before—he didn't seem to have the organization for it. He hadn't been able to let his spine curve at the top, the way dogs generally arch upward to get those back legs under them.

During this time I was pretty vigilant when we went to the dog park to avoid any kind of interaction with a dog that looked like it might be too rough with him—try to mount, put any extra pressure on his back quarters or cause him to have to run away—because he was doing an odd protective run whenever another dog would come up in an aggressive way. Clancy's back legs would stiffen, and I don't think it was necessarily about the relationship between the two dogs. It didn't look like the kind of stiffening where they are telling each other, "that's not okay with me." It was more like a protective way to use both back legs to step forward at the same time instead of alternating, and I tried to avoid those situations so he didn't re-injure himself. I think he did stress the ACL injury a couple of times, and we would notice him favoring or limping a little bit. My husband and I watched him closely to see if he was limping, and for awhile we did see it fairly often. Then slowly, some time after the third session, the limping seemed to pass.

I went back to the third session with less of an interest in organizing his movement and more of an interest in whether there was some kind of doggy psychological piece involved. I was curious about whether he was reacting to aggression by that stiffening because he doesn't have self-confidence. That sounds really funny for a dog, but it seemed as though he didn't have confidence in his movement. During the third session he started to vocalize, doing what seemed to be a practice "grrrrr!"

He didn't seem angry at us and we played it up a little bit to let him feel that response. Briah was giving him some suggestions, almost like hypnotic suggestions, which she's found very effective when animals are in more of an altered state. She talks with them about how powerful they are, that they are confident, etc., and we did some of that with Clancy.

I had brought a chewy toy, a bully stick, to this session and part of me was wondering whether I should let him have it. Clancy was chewy-chew-chewing on it so intently that he almost lost himself, and kept making his "arrr-arrr-arrr" noise. I wondered if this was getting in the way of the Rolfing, but it felt like he needed to chew, and it seemed like he was finding or releasing something through that, finding confidence. He wasn't being protective of it, rather he was really integrating his chewing movements and his body movements—or something like that. I know that with children who have problems with fine motor skills, that often there is an oral component to it. They need to do a lot of mouth and

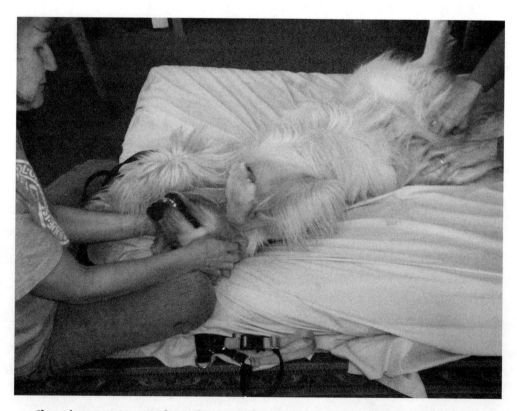

Clancy's owner, Anne and I working together as I do some deep abdominal work to better connect his hind legs to his pelvis.

hand coordination in order to get nerve pathways in their brain to flourish and myelinate. So we just let Clancy keep chewing and "aarr"-ing. He was kind of snotty at that session as I recall, and we called it off early.

It's been about six months now since the Rolfing, and Matt and I were talking the other day about whether we'd seen any evidence of Clancy favoring the leg. Neither of us had seen him limping for a long time. The jury is still out as to whether he will have issues later on, whether arthritis will set in, or anything similar that the vets were warning us about if we didn't do the surgery. But my sense is that his injury was exacerbated by not having organization in his hind legs early on, and the physics of the joints weren't working the way they were supposed to. Now that they are better aligned, his movement is a lot less stressful and I feel like we won't see these other problems develop.

Observations and Questions

I remember mentioning to Briah during the second session, that it seemed like he was getting stronger in his back end. It seemed as though his muscle mass had started to increase, like the circulation that was feeding the muscles in his back legs improved so that he could build muscle. Or perhaps it was better metabolism or just plain exercise and being able to use all of his muscles in a more balanced way. Briah told me that Rolfing does actually build up the tissues, so it is not unusual to see animals or people with atrophied muscles start becoming stronger and develop muscle mass.

The other piece that I found fascinating, and I remember talking with Briah about this even in the first session, was that the Rolfing I was doing myself was addressing mobility in my hips and an area there that I always thought was a bone. Briah said, "Whoa, this is really hard back here, and it's supposed to be soft," and she worked to bring that back to normal. I know children pattern after the adults in their lives, and I thought, "Oh, so my dog is patterning after me." I wondered if Clancy's releasing of the holding in his hip area was happening in parallel with what I was releasing at the same time. I don't know how much to read into that, but who else do puppies have to pattern after once they've left their mothers?

Clancy is a service dog, and that leads me to the one last question that I have about him, which is that I still feel that it is uncomfortable for him to sit. In our work together it is often expected that he sit. I don't think that his discomfort is behavioral. I think that there is still something structurally amiss. Part of it is the slippery hospital floors; he is so fluffy that when he sits down his back end slides out, but even so, it would be nice if he had more comfort in sitting. He usually just lays down, and that makes it a little difficult in most hospital settings because most of the patients aren't on the floor! So it would be better if he could sit by their chair. He doesn't sit anywhere, even at home. He seems to prefer lying down, walking or standing. I don't actually know how common sitting is as a position for canines. I know it's not all that healthy a position for humans, and maybe it isn't for dogs either. Perhaps he's making a really good choice for a canine.

Another change I've seen in him since the Rolfing is that he has become more playful with other dogs and runs more. He's developed into more of a typical Golden Retriever. Before Rolfing, when we were at the dog park and someone had a ball flinger, he would start out with the other dogs, happily watching with his tongue hanging out. When they flung the ball the other dogs would take off after it, but Clancy always stayed within ten yards of us and met the dogs as they returned. Now he goes all the way out with the dogs and even gets the ball occasionally. He's not a dog that has to be the first to the ball but its fun when he does get it and he'll get all "strutty."

He gets that way in the hospital now, too. He loves the attention, everybody saying "Oh, it's Clancy!" When he's in settings where he doesn't get that attention, you can almost see him saying "Whoa, what's going on here, why isn't anyone fawning over me?" I think he now has a confidence that he didn't have before, and he's more confident with other dogs. He seems to enjoy the feeling of his kind of prance.

We dog owners all live in fear of hip dysplasia, especially with big dogs, and the long term joint problems limiting their lifespan. It makes sense to me to get ahead of it when the dog is young and make sure that they have the best in structural work and movement organization. Rolfing makes a lot of sense to me early in a dog's life to really maximize their organization, decrease wear, and build the muscles strongly from the get-go. I highly recommend it.

One thing that Briah said to me that I found really interesting to reflect on was that with dogs or cats, there are so many babies *in utero*, with so many arms and legs and a lot of crowding, that there can be a lot of opportunities for distress. A pup could appear healthy, but you just don't know how its structure or movements were compromised by pressure, what might have twisted, or what his growing capabilities were *in utero*. I thought about that, and realized that it makes a lot of sense to get those twists and pressures out when they are little and not wait for them to turn into big problems later.

A friend of mine had her dog, Annie, Rolfed. She's a very different breed from Clancy, a very different structure. What was interesting to me was how different the Rolfing experience looked for her versus Clancy. Part of the difference was in their ages, breeds, and type, but it helped me to understand Rolfing better. I realized that it isn't really a recipe, it's specific to each dog's needs—structural needs and emotional needs.

Annie had sustained a very serious injury about a year ago, and I could see in the little snippet of her Rolfing that I saw that it was a very different unfolding from Clancy's. That was stunning to me because when I think about massage it's all about relaxing muscles, and it's pretty much the same for everyone. But Rolfing is more complex than that. It's not about relaxing muscles; it's engaging with the whole physiological and emotional system, so it's going to be very different depending on injuries, congenital make-up, or what is there emotionally in the dog. All in all, it was a really fascinating experience to go through. I later sent my husband and sons in for Rolfing as well. I'm glad we did it when he was a puppy instead of when he was having difficulty as a ten-year-old. I just felt like it was the time to address it.

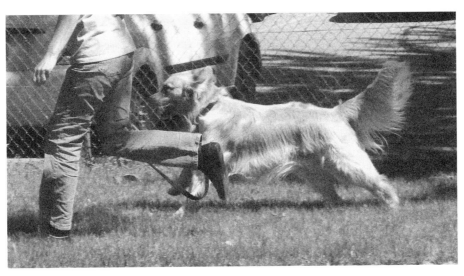

After the third session, Clancy running with a free and fully extended body.

Better than Ever: The Results of Extreme Injury

An Interview with Chris Bye and Roberta Scherf
about Annie, an English setter

Chris Bye: Annie is an English setter, almost five years old. Our Rolfing® story began last fall. I had taken Annie out pheasant hunting into some swampland and heavy grass. During the middle of the night she started panting and was obviously in pain. Normally she would jump up on the foot of the bed and sleep, but she had tremendous difficulty getting up on the bed. Once there she shook and couldn't move, and in the morning she couldn't get off the bed. From the front of her hips to the back she seemed to have a tremendous amount of pain—like her hips were locked up. I had to carry her outside where she could stand, but her feet were together. It looked like her hind quarters had stopped working and she was in a lot of pain.

I was quite distressed and took her in to the vet. The vet looked at her and walked by. He didn't seem to show a whole lot of concern as I sat there thinking my dog was going to be passing away any moment. He had Annie stand as well as she could, and he took her head and bent it right down between her front legs which caused her spine to create this tremendous arch. He massaged her head for a few seconds, and then Annie shook and went outside, went to the bathroom, and actually started to move. Not as well as before, but it indicated that it was something structural that had gone wrong. He gave her some pain meds and we took it easy and in a short amount of time she was somewhat back to normal, at least to the point where I couldn't really notice it. She seemed fine throughout the winter.

Roberta Scherf: When you brought her in, you were emailing me at four in the morning saying, "I think she's dying."

CB: She was completely immobile. This was in early December of 2008. She was in pain and she couldn't walk. She'd fall over. Her back legs were completely stiff and her paws were right near each other so she had no foundation to stand on. I had to carry her everywhere.

RS: He thought maybe there had been an injury.

CB: I think what happened is that when we were walking through the tall grass there were potholes, and she runs so fast and hard that she fell into a hole and the force of it kind of accordion compressed her spine.

RS: The vet gave Chris some exercises and said it's a physical injury. I didn't think that she would ever regain full motion and that you'd have to continue to massage her and treat the pain and discomfort.

CB: We worked at it and Annie seemed fine. This winter I took her out for a lot of walks, and as spring rolled around I did notice that she wasn't quite as smooth or energetic as she was before. I'd take her for a twenty-minute walk and she would come back tired. She had no reserves. After a walk, she'd lie down and to get going again she'd have to do a lot of stretches. I could tell that after any physical activity she was pretty cooked, and it took her awhile to stretch out enough to do what she wanted to do. Someone who didn't know the dog would think she was still very active, but compared to how she had been something wasn't quite right. She used to move more fluidly, but after the injury it looked to me like her back and her front were fused from being so tight. She seemed shorter, and the fluidity in her gait and stride was just not the way it had been. I just had this overriding concern that something was wrong.

RS: Her personality seemed a bit shorter as well. She just didn't have the equanimity, you know, the grace.

CB: She was a happier dog before the injury, much more carefree.

Annie's First Session

CB: Roberta recommended Briah to me through her friend, Anne Schuerger. We knew Anne had taken her pup, Clancy, to Briah and since this was a physical injury, it seemed like a natural to work with Rolfing. Annie is very attuned to energy as well, so it seemed like another reason to try the Rolfing. There was a real energy connection with Briah. It was not just someone going in and manipulating her, it was how the person was doing it and who the person was that made the big difference.

RS: The first session was hilarious because just a few minutes into the session all of a sudden there was this spiral unwinding and Annie just unwound into what Briah was doing. We were surprised first of all that she would even sit for the whole thing, or that she would respond so well and not try to just get out of there. But it seemed like she knew that Briah was giving her what she needed.

CB: She actually leaned into Briah in positions that I hadn't seen her in before. It looked like as Briah was working into her, Annie was working toward her trying to get as deep as possible. I think she was actually enjoying it. The first thing I noticed is that as she was being Rolfed all of a sudden her head popped up. Instead of her head being forward, her head

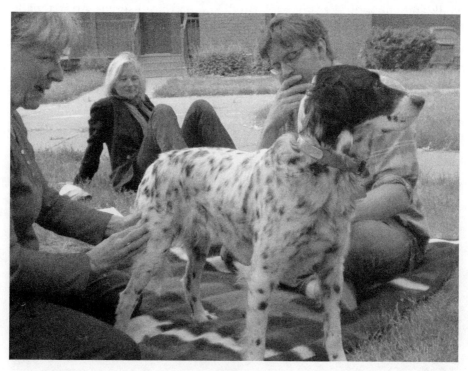

Chris Bye (Annie's owner) and Roberta Scherf (Annie's part-time guardian), look on as Annie, a five-year-old year old English setter, experiences her first Rolfing® SI session.

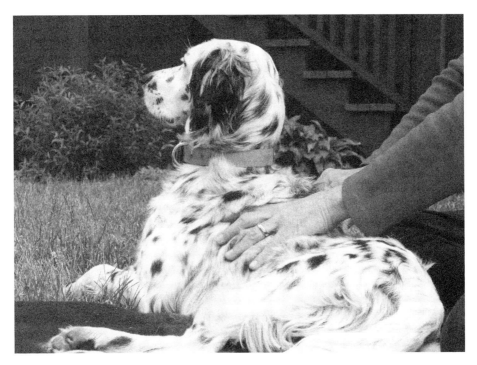

Afte three sessions, Annie is proudly coming into herself.

popped up and out. It was in a vertical line again which we hadn't seen for awhile. All of a sudden she just became more vertical and stretched out.

Fluidity and Energy

RS: The first session was more visibly transformational than any others because it was very dramatic—we could see it happen during the session. When she got up to move afterward she had gained inches—there was a lengthening and a relaxation . . .

CB: . . . and a fluidity had returned to her gait. I could see her front and her back move independently, instead of like when you have a bad back: your walk is very tight and you expend a lot of energy trying to keep everything together because if it goes out, it's painful. It was like the pain had released and she could allow her back half to move one way and the front half to move the other way. This ease in her gait came back. I would say that 90 percent of the improvement we could see came after that first session.

RS: The other two sessions (all three were about a week apart) sort of cemented and anchored the work that Briah had done in the first one. After the first session she also became happy again. She is with other dogs during the day, and she was "shorter" with them before the Rolfing. But when she was able to relax into things again, she seemed to have reserves.

CB: She ran around the house multiple times that night after the first session, doing her quick turns. She was herself again. She has a really stupid expression when she is happy. She sits there with her tongue halfway out and this silly doggy smile. That came back, and we had not seen that in a while, remember?

RS: She is also a really intelligent dog but part of the intelligence has to do with the fact that she is kind of a practical joker and a trickster, and she operates at a really high level of canine intelligence.

CB: Yeah, she used to instigate play, not only with people but with other dogs. She had stopped doing that because of the pain, but it came back as well.

RS: She started making a lot more eye contact again. She's a dog who does a lot of eye contact. If you're in the house with her, she will follow you, she'll make eye contact and she'll communicate through her eyes. She had been doing that but after Rolfing she really came into full bloom, and she is now healthier than she's ever been in her whole life.

CB: Her fatigue left. After she goes for a run she'll sit there with a big smile on her face now instead of escaping to sleep. She acts like she's ready to go again, and it seems like her energy has doubled.

RS: Tremendous energy reserves, yeah.

Personality and Behavior

CB: Annie has always been a bit protective and she had a pretty traumatic puppyhood so I'd always been a bit careful with her in certain situations. She was five months old when I got her and she came from a really terrible situation. The guy had puppies that he didn't expect and he was a backyard breeder. Her parents were beautiful dogs, but when I found Annie she was in a kennel with eight other puppies of the same age and there was—I'm not exaggerating—a foot and a half of dog poop on the kennel floor, and she was brown. I had to give her three baths to get her white and black again. She was not socialized at all well. I actually rescued two dogs from that kennel group, but we had to put the other dog down within three weeks because it was so skittish and scared of people that there was no possibility of rehabilitation.

RS: She hadn't been socialized and the kennel situation was abusive in terms of being too small and just not well cared for. She's always been guarded and she became really protective, especially around Chris, because he was like her salvation. When she's with him, she's on alert and very guarded. But she has also been really, really terrified of thunderstorms and different things. Before she came to see Briah or started her homeopathic remedy, she would stay at my house sometimes but would not sleep on the bed. She would look for a corner and I'd make a protective little pillow nest for her, but even that would be too scary. So sometimes I would just sit up with her and she'd sit in my lap shaking.

CB: She's not a passive dog at all. When you meet her, she's not at all a shy demure dog. She carries herself quite confidently. She is not gunshy. Most loud noises don't scare her except for thunder and fireworks, which I don't think is unusual for dogs. But we did give her a homeopathic remedy and that made a difference. Within a couple weeks of giving her the remedy, I had her at a cabin in the woods with the windows open during a big thunderstorm. Instead of trying of escape to the side of the bed or the closet, she sat at the foot of the bed and looked out the window and just sat there, observing the storm instead of running from it. I'm not saying she loved it, but it was definitely a different experience. She wasn't happy, but the nervousness wasn't there and it was a much different response than she'd ever had.

RS: She did the same thing at my place. We had a thunderstorm one night and she didn't even get out of bed, she just laid there. The other two dogs, of course, were getting a little bit skittish and nervous but not Annie. It was as though the level of anxiety and fearful anticipation had quieted down, and she just waited for the storm to pass. While she's been at my house there are often other dogs around, as well as delivery men, lots of people and partying, and she's been very comfortable with all of it. I haven't seen any aggression or anxiety at all. She's become more even-tempered and calm since the Rolfing and homeopathy. Three months later, she's a really happy dog.

An Optimal State of Health

CB: She gets to run a lot. Everyday I take her down to the river and let her run on the trails and in pastures. I take her grouse hunting and she loves to run in the woods. I just noticed again that she was tightening up a little bit. Maybe part of it is because she has become much more muscular, more solid, and so maybe the muscles have built up and she moves differently. I thought she was muscular in the spring; but she's gotten stronger, even more muscular since the Rolfing. I think she has lost some of the fluidity, and looks like she is fighting her run a little. I thought that with the hunting season starting up and all the running exercise she's going to be getting, I'd get another Rolfing session for her so she's as agile and mobile as she can be.

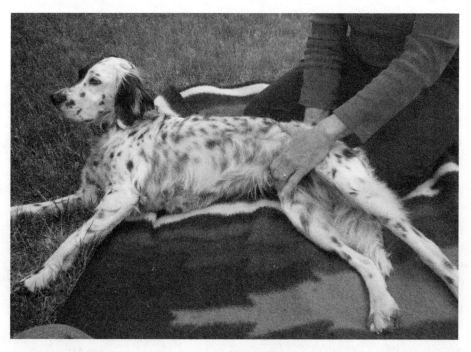

My work with Annie helped her go from immobility and pain to fluidity, agility, and freedom.

RS: She didn't look like she was in pain but to see her now after this last session, she doesn't look like a five-year-old dog, she looks like a two- or three-year-old dog: very effortless.

CB: After today's session, her gait just loosened up again. She looks longer again and she's moving her front and her back hips independently. There is this fluidity and ease of movement.

RS: Flexibility. She can undulate. She moves very gracefully and very easily, like water.

CB: Much different. I like seeing that. She was tense and compacted and now she is lengthened and released, if that makes sense. I'll probably bring her back throughout the season because she runs a lot and sometimes falls in holes or runs into a log. She's moving fast in very weird circumstances. I think I'm a little hyper-aware now since her last injury that might have resulted in something really debilitating if she hadn't been Rolfed. I watch her more closely now for signs that she's getting tight again, and will take her in for Rolfing whenever she needs it.

I brought her in to the vet three weeks ago to get her shots and a checkup. He's a really progressive vet and I told him about the Rolfing, what it had done and how she seemed really healthy. He didn't ask me questions about the Rolfing, which I was hoping he would, but he did say that she was probably the healthiest dog they had seen in a long time. They said she is just absolutely dead-on healthy. It's nice to get that feedback.

There are all kinds of options for dogs with injuries or joint problems. The Rolfing is my choice of therapies for physical injuries. I think there is a time and place for everything but I will always consider a session of Rolfing to see what happens. Dogs are different than people: they don't have this consciously preconceived notion of what's going on, they just bring things in. I would strongly recommend taking a dog in for a Rolfing session and judge the results yourself.

Birds of Prey

Briah talks about her introduction to working with raptors

The following stories are about a golden eagle, Cinnabar, and a great horned owl, Rufus. They arise from my personal recollections augmented by review of the videotaped sessions we made for documentation.

The opportunity to work with Cinnabar came from a client of mine, Dennis Ammerman. He had been training for a triathlon event, and after a few sessions he realized that his running, biking and swimming were greatly improved, and his muscle strength and performance had been greatly enhanced. Dennis had been working at a petting zoo in Overland Park, Kansas, and in particular had been working for about six months with a golden eagle that had been shot through the right wing, up through his right eye (resulting in loss of the eye), and out through the top of his head. As a result of this serious injury, he had not been able to fly to the glove very well.

My interest in working with an eagle came with some trepidation because I was worried or fearful that he might take a nibble out of my hand or arm. I saw this venture as an opportunity to apply the principles of Rolfing® Structural Integration to the animal kingdom. The tremendous success I was having with human clients gave me hope that it could restore function and dignity for these birds of prey.

Cinnabar and Rufus were the very first birds I had ever worked with. My work was not coming from specific knowledge of bird anatomy; rather from an understanding of the anatomy of form, and how structure translates into appropriate function, (i.e., movement). I saw wings as relating to the arm/shoulder girdle structure and how that connects to the entire body of the bird. Applying the principles of Rolfing SI, I worked to relate all the layers of tissue from surface to middle to deep, to give balance to both sides of the body, and to establish a midline down the center of the bird, through the head and neck and the body, and to be able to see the legs directly under the body of the bird with a nice vertical lift from the perch.

I did three sessions with Cinnabar over the course of a month's time, each lasting one to one and a half hours. The story that Dennis tells reveals the story of Cinnabar's progress. For me, this was a thrilling experience and one that would give me more confidence in my ability to rehabilitate any bird species.

Dennis Talks about Rolfing® SI and Cinnabar

In my very first session of Rolfing, the first thing I noticed that surprised and impressed me was that my lung capacity increased between 15 and 20 percent. I was really amazed because I was in good shape. I had been doing triathlons and was having tightness in my legs which would occur about fifteen to twenty miles into a bike ride. There were a number of things besides my leg that were affected, but that was the most obvious thing. I started seeing changes in my legs after the third or fourth session.

I broke my back six or seven years ago. The break caused a 65 percent compression fracture. The vertebrae could not sit on a horizontal plane. They became twisted, so I had a very deep curvature of the spine. I couldn't sit straight. I would slouch after only a few minutes of trying to sit up. Since the Rolfing, there is a substantial difference. I feel stronger.

In the past when I ran, my feet slapped the pavement. It was very hard for me to land softly on my feet no matter how hard I would try. It was uncomfortable. Now, about a year after the Rolfing, it's very easy to run. My feet land where they are supposed to.

I've not only found Rolfing to be very beneficial to me and my body, but I have also seen the same type of benefit for birds of prey. Anything with muscle tissue can benefit from Rolfing.

Early in the summer, I began working with birds of prey at a petting zoo, among them a male golden eagle named Cinnabar that had been shot. The shot was apparently from beneath the bird while it was roosting. The shot affected a little bit of wing, the main joint on the wrist, and it went through the right side of the skull. With Cinnabar, I was curious to see how depth perception was affected with just one eye. I found there was very little change when he flew from the air to the fist. He seemed to land as well with one eye as with two.

This nine-year-old bird had never been handled with human hands. Basically a wild bird, he had been kept in a cage without handling. I started working with the bird, putting some jesses on it. Jesses are the leather bracelets around the ankles so the bird can be kept close to the handler. The bird can be taken outside without worrying about it flying off. It's on a leash just like a dog would be.

I worked with Cinnabar about an hour every day. My objective was to get him outside so that people could see him fly. Some days I would get him to fly to the fist fairly easily. He would go three or four days before

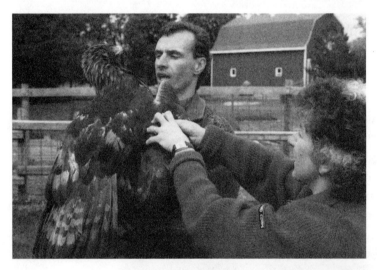

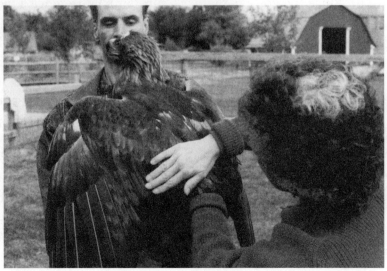

During my second session with Cinnabar he relaxed and opened his feathers like a cape and remained this way for the rest of the hour. Photos by George Terril.

he was ready to fly to the fist again. I was using food as the key to training, but eagles can eat a lot of food at one time and then they won't get hungry for four or five days after feeding.

My long-term goal was to get Cinnabar to fly to the glove consistently enough that I could release him to hunt normal prey, such as rabbits, snakes, and mice. My hopes and aspirations were to release the bird back to the wild. I had been working with the bird about five months when I mentioned the experience to Briah during my regular Rolfing session.

Cinnabar and Rolfing® SI

Briah had Rolfed a couple of Thoroughbred jumping horses, as well as a couple of Quarter Horses. I thought it would be interesting to see what kind of results would occur with a bird. When I initially proposed it, Briah was a bit hesitant. Cinnabar was a very wild bird. When I would stroke the bird's neck he would always attempt to bite me.

I didn't know what would happen or how Cinnabar would respond to being touched. I decided to construct a makeshift hood because I didn't have one large enough to fit him.

There's usually no reason to hood an eagle. Hooding basically calms the bird because he cannot see. I wanted a hood that would work so when Briah started Rolfing him, he wouldn't get too excited and bite or claw. The hood didn't work very well, so we decided to try Rolfing him without it to see what would happen.

When I work with a bird, I have a very large multilayered leather gauntlet that I made for my left hand. The bird sits on that. The arm is covered about halfway up, five or six inches above the elbow. On my other hand, the hand I would use to feed the bird, I would wear a large welder's glove which is very thick.

For safety and to try to ensure the best opportunity to actually Rolf the bird, I placed my gloved hand and arm on Cinnabar's perch and then had him stand on my glove. Next, I took his jesses and pulled them tight under my hand so he couldn't "foot" Briah. The feet are the most dangerous part of a bird of prey. The power of the talons going through the spinal column is strong enough to kill a dog. I'm nervous around even smaller birds, such as red-tailed hawks, which weigh maybe a pound and a half. The red-tail can go through several layers of glove and a quarter inch into the skin. Cinnabar weighs more than nine and a half pounds and is about eighteen inches tall with a wingspan of six- to six-and-a-half feet.

When Briah started with Cinnabar, she approached the bird from the back. I think she wanted to be as far away from his head as possible. She went behind the bird and underneath the wings into his body. I was immediately surprised. Cinnabar is very nervous and usually turns immediately to face the person. He didn't do that. He didn't even turn his head around!

When she first made contact, Cinnabar extended both wings and made a loud sound. Briah kept her hands on the bird to maintain control and immediately started Rolfing. It was about fifteen minutes before Cinnabar even looked at her. Any time I would stroke his feet, whether he was on my fist or a perch, he would immediately look down to see what I was doing. He's a very sensitive bird. Since he didn't do that while Briah was working with her hands underneath both his wings, I was surprised. He finally looked around very calmly and acknowledged that Briah was there. He looked back around as if it were just as natural as could be. After a few minutes, he began to calm down, making this frequent "chirping" sound, which he does sometimes when I am around him with food and after he has just eaten. He doesn't do it frequently. However, during the entire two-hour session, he continued to make this sound. It was a very calming sound. I don't know if there is a term for it. His beak was partially open and his tongue was hanging out a bit. It's like a very relaxed talking.

I noticed that after about ten to fifteen minutes, the bird started to relax. He started to recline toward Briah, even though he was still fully supporting his weight and had his feet in a very powerful grip. This state of relaxation lasted for the first thirty minutes. His legs were nearly on a horizontal plane but still totally supporting his weight. At that point, I realized I didn't have to worry about him "footing" Briah or being aggressive.

Cinnabar was very much in an altered state, relaxing and going with the Rolfing. Sometimes Briah would get into a painful part on the wing or body where he had been injured. The bird would almost "wake up" even though his eye was open. He'd make a high-pitched shrill noise indicating his pain and irritation. It was as if Briah hit a sore spot while working on a client and they let her know it's very tender. Cinnabar even flapped his wings a bit. But within a minute or two he was back in the same position, laying back but still gripping and holding himself in a horizontal position.

Briah was struck by the massive and multilayered musculature of this nine-and-a-half-pound bird. She said that at times it almost felt like she was working on a horse. During the session, I could see how the bird began to relax. His eye was not focused. It was a distant stare, very calm, very relaxed. Several times we would have to reposition him because it was difficult for Briah to bend over for long periods of time. The perch was about two feet tall. The bird was about eighteen inches above that. So about forty-five minutes into the session, I picked Cinnabar up on my arm and Briah worked on him at her shoulder level. Within a few minutes, he was very relaxed and started lying down against me. I had to support him with my chest because he was leaning against me as if he wanted to lie down. Again, these birds never lie down. The only time they do is in a nesting environment. They sleep upright, they stand upright, all day long and all night long. They never lie down. So when he did, I was a little surprised.

We progressed down and Briah started working on his legs. Cinnabar would have had easy access to Briah's hand if he wanted it. As she worked, he didn't even look down. When she worked on the back of his neck, right up at the top, he put his head down as if he were guiding her. He was very much in tune with the whole process.

At one point, he lay down on the glove next to my body and his right wing was totally re-laxed, fully extended, hanging from the glove down past my knees. It was like a cape of feathers. Briah grabbed the wing and started lifting it to work on it, extending it and so forth. The bird behaved as if he were sedated, something more akin to what one would ex-pect from a pet chicken rather than a powerful bird of prey. If I had moved my hand in front of him, he would not have acknowledged it. And remember, this was a wild bird, very alert, very keen. I was amazed. It was beautiful.

Every fifteen or twenty minutes, Cinnabar would appear to wake him-self up, analyze the situation, and within a minute or two get back into the altered state again. When Briah was working under his wings she re-marked how his wings were almost like a shade. She extended his wing over the top of her so she could see underneath.

We progressed down and Briah started working on his legs. Cinna-bar would have had easy access to Briah's hand if he wanted it. As she worked, he didn't even look down. When she worked on the back of his neck, right up at the top, he put his head down as if he were guiding her. He was very much in tune with the whole process. Briah said that Cinnabar seemed much more appreciative than some of the other animals she had worked with, even though the others had been domestic.

I remembered that every time I got out of a Rolfing session, one of the very first things I would have to do is eat. Even if I had eaten an hour before I went in, I was famished. Thinking that it might be the same with Cinnabar, I fed him right after the session.

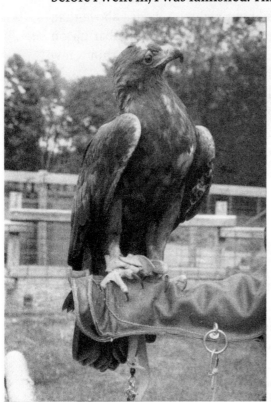

After three sessions Cinnabar stands tall and proud.

Briah then suggested that we have Cinnabar fly to the glove a few times. I told her I would try. However, since he had just eaten, it might be two or three days before he would eat again. I might not be able to get him to fly. He flew three or four times to the glove, which surprised me. I noticed that he landed more softly than he had before. In the past, he would land at the same speed at which he was flying. Other birds I had worked with would use their wings in a braking method, their tails fully fanned. This was the first time he had done it right in the six months I had worked with him. This was about thirty minutes after the Rolfing session.

In analyzing the pictures, I noticed Cinnabar was more balanced. The left side looked more like the right side. He used to look as if he had bowed legs. One leg went further up into the body and that side of the body seemed turned and twisted a bit. The neck and head were rather short, shrunken into the shoulders. After Rolfing, the rest of his body looked fuller, more rounded and filled out. It was as if he had grown two or three sizes. His weight hadn't changed, but he looked as though he'd gained a few pounds from the way his body had expanded.

Cinnabar's neck was larger, fuller, taller. This bird is very powerful. When he flies, his wings should be fully extended, but prior to the Rolfing he could not manage full extension. The photographs are quite dramatic. They show the improved power of flight after the Rolfing session.

About a month later, Briah did another Rolfing session with Cinnabar. During that month, he hadn't seemed quite as frightened. He had more confidence. Before, Cinnabar seemed rather timid and weak, not only in his physical body, but also in his overall posture. It was noticeable in the way he carried himself and the way he stood on his perch.

He learned—probably relearned—how to slow down in flight and stop. Previously, he would land on my fist at full speed, knocking me back a step or two. His mass of nine and a half pounds combined with his momentum forced me to hold my gloved fist overhead to avoid having his wings hit me in the face and head. Cinnabar has a lot more control over his body now. He is more coordinated, more like a bird from the wild would be. They can land softly on anything. There was a gracefulness that he regained. Before the Rolfing, he would come in for a crash landing. The first time or two that he flew to the glove at a distance of six to eight feet, I had to step back to regain my balance because there was so much force and energy coming toward me. During the months after he was Rolfed, Cinnabar would come in and slow down, landing right on that spot. I wouldn't have to take a step backward.

When we did the second session, it was videotaped by a local TV station. It was a very windy day. With the lifting strength of these birds, it was difficult to hold onto Cinnabar's leash. He would hover right above the glove about two or three inches. It was like flying a kite. The wind constantly threw him off balance. So we moved to work with him around the side of the barn.

Briah seemed more relaxed, having worked with him before. It seemed to take only a few minutes for Cinnabar to get into that altered state again. He recognized Briah, just like he recognized me. He was very calm and relaxed. I didn't have him on the perch. He lay down several times during that session which lasted a couple of hours. We reworked those areas where the injury had occurred. Briah was able to do some very specific work in between the joints in the right wing and through the entire wing.

The structure of the wing is similar to a person's arm. Imagine bringing your wrist up next to your shoulder. Your wrist and shoulder represent the thick mass you see on a bird's wing when it's folded. The other part of the elbow is actually back below the softer tissue that makes a slight "U" shape from the shoulder to the elbow. When you extend that, the tissue extends as well, stretching and actually covering the elbow that's now extended.

The first time Briah worked with him, she didn't do much with that area. It was very tense and tight. She spent a lot of time freeing up that entire wing structure during the second session. Cinnabar was able to relax and allow her to work in those very sensitive areas. Once when she was working on him there, a muscle in his wing twitched and quivered. He was again in an altered state. Briah was able to get deeper. A friend of ours put her hands on Briah's hands. She could feel some of the tissue releasing. I was holding the bird upright to keep him from falling off. By this time, he was lying down, which is very unnatural for these birds.

We had problems getting him to stand back up a couple of times. He was so into the altered state that he didn't want to finish the session. We had to stand him back up so Briah could work on his chest and legs some more. She even kissed the back of his head because she was so comfortable with him.

Before this session, I noticed that Cinnabar's eye was looking really dry. During the session, it started to look shinier, a little more oily. The eye was able to rotate in the socket better. After Briah Rolfed Cinnabar, we decided to try it on an owl.

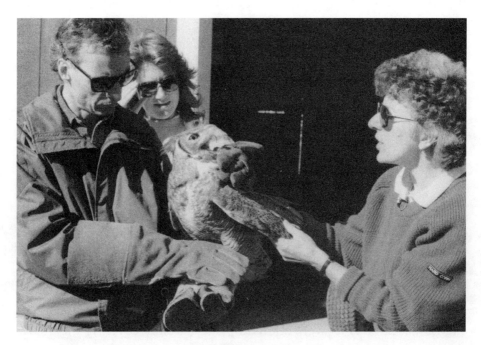

I'm carefully negotiating the territory with Rufus. Photo by George Terril.

Briah Talks about Rolfing® SI and Rufus

Rufus was a nine-year-old great horned owl who had been hit by a car, resulting in a dislocation of his jaw. He had received surgical care and some repairs were attempted to correct the dislocation, but not enough to allow Rufus to eat roadkill. After this accident, Rufus did not have the ability to tear meat apart; consequently, he was fed a diet of ground meat. Because of this severe injury, it was clear to the veterinarians that Rufus would never be able to survive in the wild.

The Rolfing® SI session that I did with Rufus was an experiment and an exploration to see if it would be able to change the severely overlapping beak. I worked my way carefully and in an exploratory way, finding musculature that was too tight or bound up and then freeing it so that there was more resilience and freer movement.

I proceeded initially with Rufus by making contact from behind the body. I was not interested in having this bird bite me, so that was the reason for working from behind. I worked my way up through the back of Rufus' body, freeing the connections of the wings to the body, then continuing through the neck and the head.

As with classic TMJ (temporomandibular joint syndrome), typically it's an issue of the cranium not fitting the jaw, so I did as much work as I could on the outside of Rufus' neck and head. Finally, with the aid of Dennis and another gloved handler stabilizing Rufus' beak from either side, I was then able to use a smaller glove and go inside his beak and mouth and completely finish aligning the jaw to itself. This was a very dramatic part of the Rolfing process as there was movement that resulted in being able to align his beak.

Within a week of this first session with Rufus, I was told that he was finally able to eat whole mice and rats. A year later I was told that he was still able to eat whole game and was doing great. This single Rolfing session resulted in a dramatic recovery and I would call it a great success story. This session gave me the confidence to work with other birds of prey and my clients' pet birds over the next twenty years.

Dennis Talks about Rufus's Rolfing® SI Session in 1989

Rufus had been injured when he flew in front of a car five or six years ago. His jaw had been broken and he couldn't pull meat apart because the lower mandible was about a half-inch left of the upper mandible. We maintained him on a diet of ground entrails, meat and bones, which is very similar to an owl's natural diet.

These meals aren't as good as live or freshly killed prey, but Rufus was not capable of pulling anything apart. He could not grab prey with his beak because it overlapped so much. It was very thin, almost like a fingernail. Two surgeries had been performed on his beak; Rufus had the best surgical care an owl could receive. When the veterinary school realized he couldn't survive in the wild, they gave him to the zoo for display and educational purposes.

The problem with Rolfing this owl was his natural instinct to bite. He's ornery. Briah would approach him from the back side and he would nip her. We finally got a fairly thin pair of leather gloves after she had worked on him as much as possible without them. He bit on a piece of the leather glove like a pacifier, watching what was going on. As long has he had something in his mouth, Rufus seemed to be somewhat content to let Briah work with him. He wasn't as cooperative as Cinnabar, the golden eagle, had been. Briah wasn't able to work with him as in-depth. She worked with his wings and with his body a little. However, Rufus didn't require as much work as Cinnabar. There wasn't as much mass to work with.

Owls have two sets of eyelids. They have eyelids from the side that actually go toward the beak at a right angle. The other set closes from top to bottom. Sometimes Rufus would close one eyelid. Sometimes he would close both. At other times he would close both eyelids on both eyes. He made little sounds. With the piece of leather in his mouth, he thought he was in full control.

After a while, Briah wanted to work with his jaw. This presented a problem since he had a piece of leather in his jaw as a pacifier. Briah used a glove to protect her hands and worked inside Rufus' mouth, trying to get the cranium to better fit the mandible. The changes we saw were amazing. It appeared that the alignment of the beak had changed substantially. It had moved three-eighths of an inch. At that point, the right side of his lower mandible would touch the upper right side of his upper mandible. Before, the two mandibles looked like a pair of scissors which were wide open.

I had not realized before the session the length of his lower mandible. It was actually too long to fit below the upper mandible properly. It occurred to me that, after the session, we were going to have to clip the lower mandible because it's supposed to fit under the upper mandible.

When Briah worked with Rufus's mouth, he made chirping noises. Occasionally, I saw him swallow. At times, it sounded like he was chirping bloody murder. His eyes were saying "don't stop." It was very entertaining, very funny. There was no struggling at all. There was no one holding the bird.

Since the Rolfing, his instinct to bite is not as pronounced as it was before. He seems more calm and less agitated. When a friend of mine works with him, Rufus doesn't seem to want to bite as often. He doesn't want to protect himself as much as before.

Rufus can now take small rodents in his talons, then tear and pull them apart with his beak. There was no way he could do this prior to the Rolfing work because his beak was so far off. It's a lot better for him to eat more of his normal prey. When an owl holds prey with their feet and pulls it apart, it strengthens the back muscles. It's good exercise, and it helps keep the beak from being overgrown. Feeding Rufus something that's ground up doesn't allow him to stretch those muscles or keep that beak in proper shape. Filing, or coping, a bird's beak is required when they're maintained on an improper diet.

Working with the face or beak requires two strong people to hold the bird completely stationary. If those powerful feet get loose for an in-

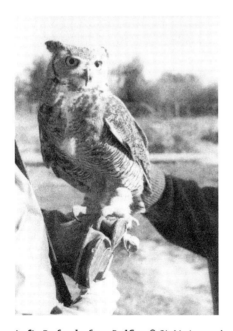 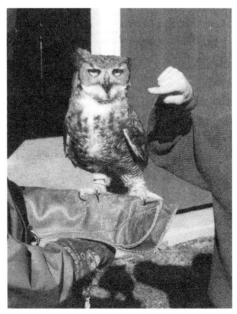

Left. *Rufus before Rolfing® SI: Note major beak misalignment.* **Right.** *After just one Rolfing® SI session I was able to get Rufus's beak aligned.*

stant, they can grab an arm and they don't let go. The talons are thrust deep into the flesh and they are needle sharp. At the same time, the bird is trying to bite. It's a huge ordeal. So the Rolfing work was relaxed compared to the ordeal of filing a beak down.

The reason for working on Rufus was to see if we could get the mandible to move. And it did—dramatically!

There are other animals and other situations in which Briah and I would like to try some Rolfing, just to see what happens. We are going to document this. Of all the animals in the animal kingdom, birds probably have the least amount of muscle tissue. I want to try a more massive animal in order to see what happens with an animal that's healthy. The next animal we're going to try working with is a mountain lion. He is about two years old and perfectly healthy. If you can find a Rolfer who's willing to work on an animal that's injured, I suggest you do it. It's definitely worthwhile.

I suggested the Rolfing work for these animals after seeing and feeling the changes I experienced. That's what this book is about. It's a compilation of stories and experiences Rolfees have had, and it's something everyone should have done.

I've referred some twenty friends and relatives for Rolfing work. Their stories are all different. Perhaps some not as dramatic as mine, but still very positive. Many of them have sent their friends because Rolfing works and they are feeling healthier. Obviously, I recommend it.

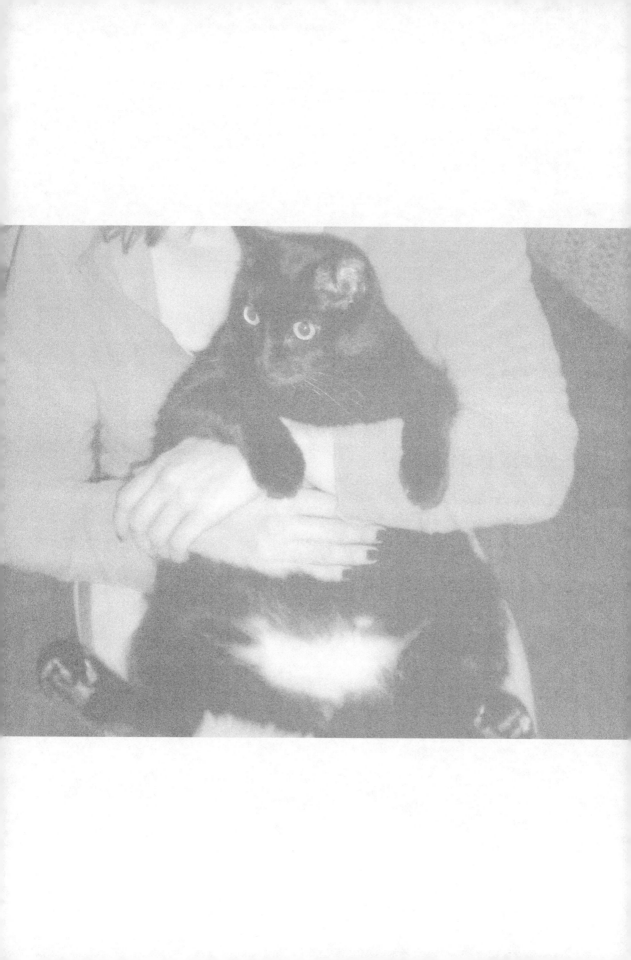

Behavior Changes
and Essence Unleashed

▶ *Rolfing is an ongoing process that continues long after the work has been completed.*

▶ *So many therapists are striking at the pattern of disease instead of supporting the pattern of health. Rolfers are not practitioners curing disease, they are specialists in health. They are giving their attention to the better working of people's minds and bodies.*

▶ *We are all looking for a way to evoke human potential. We are all looking for a way to establish greater physical and mental vitality.*

DR. IDA P. ROLF, from *Ida Rolf Talks about Rolfing and Physical Reality*, Rosemary Feitis, ed., Harper Row: NY; 1978

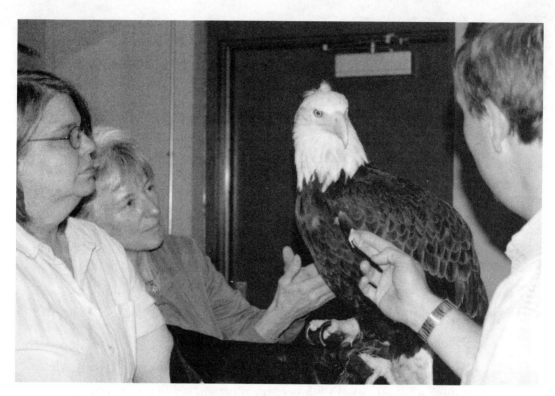

Scott Mehus, Education Coordinator at the National Eagle Center, distracts Harriet with some fresh fish as I make my initial contact with Harriet. MaryBeth Garrigan, Program Director, assists by holding Harriet on the glove. Photo by Christee Donovan.

Working with Eagles:
A Return to Balance, Poise, and Pride

Briah Anson and MaryBeth Garrigan talk about
the eagles Harriet, Angel, Donald, and Columbia

On May 25, 2007, my colleague from Canada, Penny Tanner, and I were returning to St. Paul from a week of training with "Frequencies of Brilliance" in Frontenac, Minnesota. Our planned destination was a special restaurant in Pepin, Wisconsin, so we took our time and wandered into the town of Wabasha, Minnesota. We spent several hours in the town, shopping and walking around, and discovered that there is a National Eagle Center there in a fabulous new building right on the Mississippi River.

We wandered into the Eagle Center only to learn that the center was closing in fifteen minutes. The receptionist at the front desk told us to take our time as they would be there for a while doing paperwork. Penny and I excitedly went into this large room that had three mature bald eagles on perches. We sat on the floor and spent the next half hour consciously transmitting and sending energy, and establishing a connection with the eagles. At first the eagles turned their backs to us. As we continued to work with them, one by one they began fluffing out their feathers with curiosity. At one point, both Penny and I noticed that the eagle farthest away was staring at us. Simultaneously we seemed to receive the message: "What about me? I want some of that! We then became very aware of a strong energetic connection and exchange occurring between us and the three eagles.

Penny went out to the reception area and stopped to chat with MaryBeth Garrigan, the director of the Eagle Center. She told Penny that she had walked by two or three times and noticed us working with the birds, and saw that whatever we were doing seemed to be having a very positive and relaxing effect on them. Penny told MaryBeth that we were energy healers, and also explained to MaryBeth that Briah was a Rolfer™ and had worked with a variety of birds of prey for the purpose of rehabilitating them.

At that point I came out and met MaryBeth and had a conversation with her about my work with people and animals, and the benefits of this type of soft tissue work. I proposed to MaryBeth that I volunteer to work with these injured eagles. MaryBeth explained that everything that possibly could have been done medically has been done but she understood that if some tissue work were done, this would enable the eagles to be more comfortable. I agreed to return in two weeks to attempt some Rolfing® Structural Integration with one of the eagles.

It turned out that a week later a friend and I were able to return to the eagle center on a Saturday so that I could get better acquainted with the birds, or rather, so *we* could get better acquainted! It was quite interesting to me and not surprising that the eagles seemed to recognize me. I could feel this. During this visit the eagle that I would work on first, Harriet, was engaged in an educational program in another city, so she was not there that day.

The following Friday I returned to the Eagle Center with my friend and colleague, Christee Donovan. Throughout the week, I had been chanting to connect with the eagle I would be working with in order to facilitate a more receptive interaction. (I am a Nichiren Buddhist and have found the Buddhist chants to be effective support.)

The First Eagle, Harriet

When we arrived we met MaryBeth, the director, and Scott, the education coordinator, and found out that we would be working with Harriet. Harriet is the eagle with the most impaired wing and has had multiple surgeries in an attempt to salvage a good part of her left wing. She has had a partial wing amputation and has some weakness in the left leg.

MaryBeth decided that we should work in the room where the eagles have different veterinary procedures done. Harriet was facing the area with two other eagles and had a beautiful view of the Mississippi River. MaryBeth proceeded to put some special grease on the bottom of Harriet's pads where the talons are, as this is an area that can develop hot spots from the constant sitting on perches. MaryBeth asked that I stand on the opposite side of her facing Harriet and that I start by first placing my hand above her left talon.

Needless to say, this awakened a fear response in me. I have great respect for the power of an eagle's beak and this felt like an extremely vulnerable position to be in. I calmly asked MaryBeth if it would be possible for me to work from behind Harriet as my experience working with other raptors had started in this position. MaryBeth explained that it would be a very threatening position for Harriet as she would not be able to see me and know what I was doing. I took a couple of breaths and decided to open my trust of MaryBeth and Harriet and proceeded to put my hand on Harriet's left leg just above her talons. There followed a period of several minutes (which felt like hours) of a mutual negotiation of trust going on between Harriet and myself. She occasionally flapped her wings and would move away on the perch a bit. She was obviously tentative about me and what I was doing. MaryBeth explained that given all the procedures that have been administered to Harriet this would be a very different kind of touch and Harriet did not yet know that it could be a pleasant healing experience.

As the minutes progressed and my comfort level increased, I proceeded to very slowly increase the pressure on her leg about a gram at a time. It was fascinating to observe how incredibly sensitive she was. As I proceeded to apply very subtle pressure, I became aware of feeling how this work was penetrating her entire body system. At one point not very long into the session, Harriet started to reach out with her head and neck as if she were lurching forward to see something way out in the distance. It was obvious that she was already taking this small amount of frontal Rolfing work and organizing it throughout her whole body. I have observed horses doing this kind of action as well when I work on them. In short, she was taking the input and unwinding through her whole body.

I continued to gradually move up her left leg. As I got closer up her thigh, she became nervous and tried to peck at me. I pulled away before she could get to me. MaryBeth explained that even though it was counterintuitive, it would be best for me not to remove my hands from her, as this would give Harriet the idea that I was afraid (which in fact I was), and she would persist in that aggressive behavior. I had observed Harriet even pecking at MaryBeth and I saw that MaryBeth did not pull away, and noted that Harriet was not harming her. Once again, this was a new lesson for me, and a new place to have courage and trust.

I mentioned to MaryBeth that in my work with animals and people who have been injured, I typically chose to work on the side that has not been injured or traumatized, and that in fact the work transfers over to the opposite side. I have found this to be a very noninvasive and comfortable way to proceed with injured humans and animals. This helps to establish a feeling of trust and comfort. We decided to have me stand next to and behind MaryBeth, and approach Harriet from a 45-degree angle. I immediately took a sigh of relief as this was exactly how I wanted to start the session in the first place.

By that time Harriet was starting to look much more relaxed and I proceeded to work up her right leg with much more confidence and depth. At one point I had one hand on Harriet's leg and I was increasing my pressure into the tissues of the leg as I had my other hand on MaryBeth's back. The amount of heat and energy being released out of Harriet, coming through my body, and transferring to MaryBeth was so intense I felt as if I was burning up. Christee took a couple of pictures of me working with Harriet and I look completely tan in my face. This is how much energy was being released from Harriet into my body.

Someone then brought in some fresh fish. MaryBeth had the great idea to have Scott start feeding her small morsels of fish. Each time Harriet took a bite I would move higher up on her leg and sink further into her tissues. This was a great way to anchor in food with touch in a positive experience. I started using both hands and felt the fear in both me and Harriet melting away. I felt as if I could work on Harriet for hours. It had been almost an hour and MaryBeth felt as if this would be a good time to end the session as it has been a great first experience for Harriet. Prior to this, Harriet had all her weight into her bad leg and hardly any weight on the leg I was working on. MaryBeth found this amazing and also noted that Harriet was looking extremely relaxed and calm. Her feathers were relaxed and her eyes appeared glazed which is indicative of her being in a more altered state of consciousness.

Even though it had only been an hour, I felt as if I had just spent three hours working on a large horse. When I do Rolfing work on a horse there is so much energy being released out of 1,200 to 1,500 pounds of animal and that energy runs through my body. It's like an electrical system and I can feel overloaded energetically. Even though I was not working very deeply into Harriet's tissues, there was so much condensed tissue containing incredible amounts of energy and power that I was experiencing almost the same effect. Christee, who was working energetically from eight to ten feet away, also felt tired.

We Start on Angel

On our way to Wabasha for this second Rolfing session, MaryBeth called and left a message that Harriet would not be available due to the fact that she was at a very important funeral service for a Vietnam veteran whose remains had recently been found. Harriet had been requested to attend this service. (This event made national news. The son of the Vietnam vet whose remains were found was flown from Iraq to Vietnam to escort his father's remains home.)

MaryBeth said that I could try working with Angel, another eagle, but that Angel had been exhibiting a lot of aggressive behavior this week. We called the Eagle Center to let them know we were on our way and that Angel would be our three-o'clock client.

Shortly after we arrived, Angel was taken into the education room for her three-o'clock feeding which consisted of fresh rabbit meat. Apparently she'd been extremely hungry this week. Her appetite had been insatiable although her diet is strictly monitored. We sat in on the ongoing demonstration and learned how Angel sustained her injury.

Apparently baby eaglets fight ferociously for food that the parents drop into their nest. Angel fell out of the nest and fractured a wing. The wing healed but in the wrong position. She was treated at the Raptor Center in St. Paul, Minnesota and sent to the National Eagle Center in Wabasha.

During the demonstration Angel was staring directly at me with a look so piercing, it was as if I was being worked on energetically. I felt as if I was being put into a drug-altered state.

We learned during the demonstration that an eagle has seven thousand feathers. I was not too excited to hear that the talons have the power of five hundred pounds per square inch.

Knowing that it was her left wing that was injured, I suggested to MaryBeth that we go to the opposite side of Angel's body to start the work. I stood on her side where Angel was pecking on her arm. I took my time, standing calmly next to MaryBeth to allow myself to become comfortable being less than a foot away from Angel. MaryBeth placed her hand under the wing high on the leg with the idea that I would come under her hand and start my exploration of Angel. I was amazed at how quickly I was able to make contact. MaryBeth was quite surprised that Angel allowed the work to go on.

Angel exhibited some similar behavior and responses that I saw with

Harriet, such as the deep autonomic breathing, fluffing her feathers out in a relaxed manner, opening her mouth with her tongue out, eyes glazing over. Every now and then she brought herself back, would look all around the room as if to figure out where she was and establish her bearings. Occasionally she would stretch her neck and head as if trying to organize the impact of the work. At other times she would condense herself and bring her neck and head back into her body before stretching back out.

After every few minutes of work Angel would want to "bate," which looks like the eagle is flying around in a circle, connected to a leather leash. MaryBeth explained this was an eagle's way of releasing condensed energy. Angel would immediately be relaxed by this behavior and it became an opportunity for me to move deeper into her body. She defecated four or five times within an hour which seemed to express deeper levels of relaxation. We continued the work as Angel showed no signs of distress, until it became evident all of a sudden that she was becoming agitated, as if to say, "I've had enough for one day."

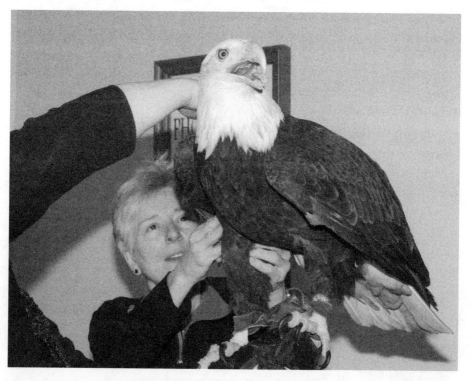

I became joyful as I felt Angel allowing me deeply into her body. I could feel her trust and acceptance as I worked with her leg.

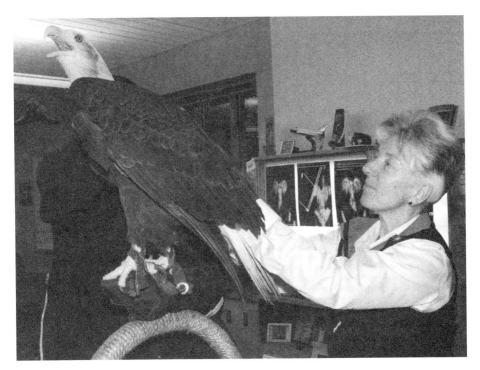

I found myself with this rare opportunity to work on both Angel's wings and their attachments to her body from behind.

MaryBeth remarked several times that Angel was releasing a tremendous amount of heat through her feet. MaryBeth talked to Angel almost continuously to assure her she was okay. She said to her frequently, "It's just you. It's just me."

I was keenly aware that Angel was just a foot away from me and every now and then would look at me directly in the eye and stare. I did a much better job of not pulling my hands away when this happened, so I would communicate to her that I too was not backing away. This seemed to deepen the trust between us so I could continue the work at a deeper level. It's as if Angel had a long conversation with Harriet describing what the Rolfing session did for her! MaryBeth said Angel goes crazy if someone other than the handlers goes near her. It struck me that it is of the utmost importance to be present every moment of this process—attempting to match these great birds and how present they were for the sessions.

(Note from an observer: I was awed that this great wild animal allowed not one but two people to touch her; one of whom was touching her deeply. After a while Angel seemed to be cooperating by lifting her wing

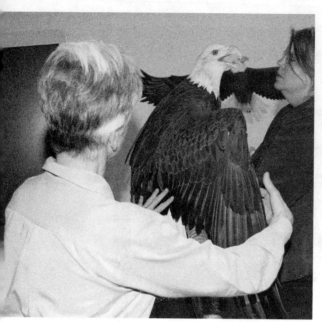

Beak open . . . softly vocalizing. Shoulders dropped. Wings falling and staying open. Ahhh! Complete relaxation of Angel.

or positioning herself a certain way. She just as easily could have bitten off both their noses or several fingers at once. I felt privileged to be there observing. *Joyce Konczyk*)

Harriet Returns For More Rolfing® Structural Integration

As of August, 2007, Harriet had a series of six Rolfing sessions. With each subsequent session it would only take a matter of two to three minutes to reestablish a hands-on connection where both Harriet and I felt mutually comfortable. I have continued to work slowly to create more space in her structure, always starting on the right side as this was her "good side." I have been working to soften and establish more balance in her tissues, i.e., from the outside to the inside of the leg, to free up her chest, loosen her up where the wing attaches to her torso and gradually working my way back toward her hind end. All of this was being done with the intention of establishing a better midline.

The reason for this (establishing the midline) was that Harriet had sustained major injuries to her body when she was struck by an automobile in 2000. Her left leg and wing were injured resulting in a partial amputation of that wing. She underwent several surgeries and hence was quite phobic about any veterinarian visits and anyone messing with her left side.

I remember noticing on my first visit that Harriet was unable to stand on her perch in a balanced way. I was told that often when she would fly from perch to perch (she has three perches) she would not be able to land successfully when the second perch was only five to seven feet away. She would frequently fall on her face. She was so unbalanced that when she would attempt to perch on the edge of her large basin of water, she would frequently fall into the basin.

After five sessions, I spoke with Scott Mehus, the full-time National Eagle Center handler of the birds. Scott reported that Harriet had been hitting the mark on her perch successfully. Now when she sits on her perch her imbalance is not noticeable. She is able to stand fairly vertical on her perch and not waver.

When I arrived on August 3, 2007, for her sixth session, Harriet was perched outside of the center sunning herself. Her right wing, which was not damaged in the car accident, was fully extended. Her left wing, more than half of which had been amputated, was also opened. Even with this weight imbalance, due to the different mass of the two wings, she was able to stand on her perch in a perfectly aligned way utilizing a tilt of her head.

Imagine drawing a line through the middle of her tail feathers which continues up through her torso to the center of her head. You would see an eagle "on her vertical line." By no means does she have equal symmetry from the left to the right side. However, because of balance established by the Rolfing sessions, Harriet is now able to find her center of gravity. One could see the value of Rolfing SI for humans who are missing limbs or parts of their body.

My first observations of Harriet showed me a bird that stood on her perch by carefully navigating her balance. She did not appear to have much confidence. MaryBeth had also told me that due to all the trauma that Harriet had sustained and her subsequent surgeries, Harriet had some arthritis and probably was in a fair amount of pain. This, of course, she would not visibly show to anyone.

One thing was clear, however; at first she did not want me to stand next to her left side. It would take until her fifth session before I was comfortable standing on her injured left side, and Harriet was comfortable having me there. This allowed me to work directly on her left leg which had also been injured in the collision. I no sooner worked for a few minutes on her left leg, finding my way to the inside of her upper leg, when she unfurled her apron of feathers. MaryBeth explained that this fluffing up of the apron feathers is an indication of complete relaxation and comfort; eagles do this in the wild to protect their young from the cold. I then worked my way up the leg to the place where her left wing attaches to her torso. Harriet continued to relax into the Rolfing touch, expanding her apron and the rest of her feathers.

This was to be a new chapter in her rehabilitation process. I felt like I'd arrived at a deeper level with Harriet and that the trust was deepening. After working for about fifteen minutes on this side it felt like a good place to terminate the session. Harriet had enough input to integrate.

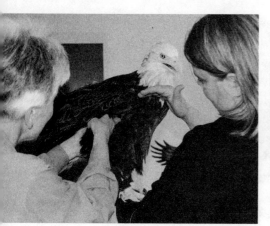 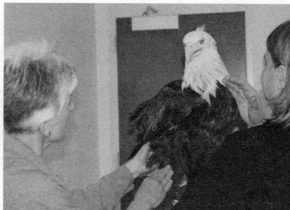

Briah is assisted by MaryBeth. An extraordinary event in eagle–human interaction: Harriet showing her trust by opening her apron of feathers—typically exhibited when protecting the young eaglets in the nest.

On August 3, for Harriet's sixth session, it literally took seconds for me to reestablish physical contact with her. I only spent about five minutes working on the right side of her body. MaryBeth and I both felt that Harriet was ready for me to work on her left side. This would only be the second time that I had even stood on her left side, let alone worked there. I immediately put my right hand where her left leg attaches to her torso. Harriet remained calm and continued to hold her head in an upright position. Had Harriet felt threatened or uncomfortable in any way she would have defended her leg by biting me with her beak.

Once I started working on the attachment of wing to torso, still on the left side, she barely looked down and actually appeared to be in an altered state. Her eyes were glazed over, her beak was open, small droplets of sweat were actually falling from her beak and from her tongue which was extended out of her mouth. MaryBeth reported that there was a tremendous amount of heat coming out of her talons. She explained that when an eagle gets hot, they perspire through their mouth. This was not heat due to stress but due to the release of energy from the Rolfing work which translates into the release of heat. This is due to the immediate increase in circulation and vascularity. We also observed an increase in space throughout the entire left side of her body. In the photograph taken from the front you can see there was an increase in mass. Harriet was beginning to look more balanced from left side to right side.

When there is soft tissue trauma, hundreds of layers of tissue become condensed and congealed. It is the job of a Rolfer™ to carefully release and create spaces in between the layers of tissue. It is in this way that we start softening fascias and repositioning muscles, tendons, ligaments and soft tissue so that the bones can migrate to more appropriate positions. The other aspect of Rolfing SI is that we do this with the intention of aligning these structures within the field of gravity. In Harriet's case this was absolutely key in helping her to find her balance point in gravity.

I worked for a total of forty-five minutes, meticulously creating space in the layers of tissue. I could feel the changes occurring. As I was working on Harriet's left side, I took a lot of breaks to look at her from the front to see the effect. I observed that she kept widening her stance and for the first time, she no longer looked bowlegged—she was actually putting equal weight on both legs. It has taken these six sessions to get Harriet to this point of balance on her two legs. We could clearly see that she was no longer struggling for balance. She was obviously much more confident and comfortable in her body.

I was just at the point of feeling complete with this session when Harriet spontaneously broke the silence. She suddenly burst into a piercing high-pitched series of vocalizations. It was one continuous sound of three to five seconds without a break. She was having a huge energetic expansion. It felt like she was using these vocalizations to express this movement of energy. Her apron fluffed and it was obvious that she was in the middle of a big release process, using these sounds as part of the release. It was also clear to all three of us that she was complete.

I felt joyful and celebratory. It gave me goose bumps. I double checked to see if she was in any distress, as did MaryBeth. Harriet was holding her head up high, her feathers were fluffed, she was proud and erect. She definitely was in no distress. At this point, I felt that with these six sessions and the alignment and balance that I witnessed, it was sufficient work for Harriet to integrate.

By integration I mean the following: I have been able to work with Harriet and help her structure find a balance point which allows her now to stand more evenly on both legs. The left and right sides of her body appear more symmetrical and she is able to maintain her neck and head over the central axis of her body. This grouping of sessions has brought Harriet's structure into a new pattern of organization. There is still more work to be done, however.

In the Rolfing system, one of the major components that we work with is how the gravitational field impacts living structures. On this planet the strongest energetic field is the field of gravity. It is a principle of Rolfing that when you align the body within the field of gravity or bring it to a new pattern of organization into the vertical, that it is important to then give the body a period of time to continue to unwind spontaneously along the vertical axis of gravity. There is an interaction between the gravitational field and the electromagnetic field. One spirals downward and the other spirals upward. It is the basic design of the double helix molecular structure that we find within each cell of the body, human or animal. Once you have brought a structure into a more organized and vertical plane, the interaction of these fields continues to unwind the cells of the body into a more vertical plane. This is what I mean by integration, and this is also what is meant by the work continuing after the work is done.

Angel Gets Her Next Rolfing® SI Sessions

One particular session with Angel that stands out for me was early on in her Rolfing process. She had had a couple of sessions and they had gone smoothly. Much to the amazement of the staff at the National Eagle Center, Angel was extremely receptive to the Rolfing work.

On this particular occasion Angel was not happy to see me. In fact, she was hissing and behaving quite ferociously. She kept trying to bite me from every direction that she could. She would go under the handler's arm and turn every which way she could to get at me. Her hackles were up and she would not stop any of her aggressive attacks. In fact, she was so worked up and had so much pent up energy she would continuously bait (fly in circles off the leather leash that was around her talons).

Her distress level was high and this was a radical departure from her previous two sessions. I was perplexed as to what was going on with Angel. She continued to try to bite me and she was clearly saying . . . "there is no way you are going to even touch me today . . . or maybe never, for that matter."

I finally remembered that Angel considered herself the Queen Diva of the eagles at the Center and it dawned on me that she was probably upset with me for working with Harriet instead of her. I decided to just step out in front of her and offer my sincere apologies. I went on and on for a couple of minutes . . . acknowledging her to be the most important eagle and also being quite contrite about my having worked with Harriet after Angel's two sessions. This seemed to calm her right down and as I sensed her energy shift to a more relaxed and calm state I stepped back to her side and asked her permission to do another session with her.

Angel just sat there on the handler's arm which was leaning on the perch and stared at me. I remembered MaryBeth's guidance which was to show Angel that I'm not afraid of her. It took all the courage I could muster to continue to hold her stare in my gaze, keep breathing, and calmly continue to invite Angel into this Rolfing partnership. With this firm determination and strong spirit I then delivered an entire hour of Rolfing work without her even attempting to bite me.

This was the most amazing session I had with any of the four eagles I worked with over that two year period. I recognized during that session that these eagles do understand what you are saying . . . or at least the energy of it. I was clearly forgiven and Angel and I moved to a new understanding. What is also significant about this event is that for the next two years I would on a weekly basis (spring through fall) work with whichever eagle seemed to be needing work the most, and Angel did not seem to care. Toward the latter part of the second year I would even work on two eagles each time I came which seemed to work quite nicely.

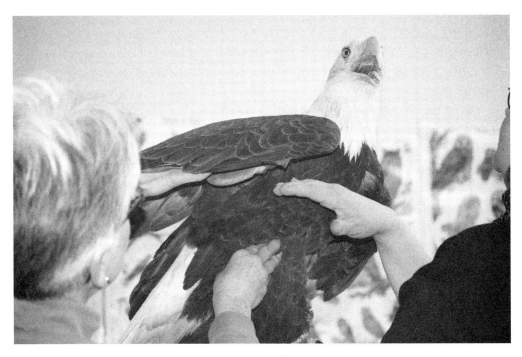

After numerous sessions with Angel, I maximize our connection.

I never had another incident with Angel where she was in this ferocious attack mode. There were times when she might be a bit agitated for five to ten minutes and try to bite at me but would settle right into the work as soon as I had my hands on her and her nervous system was able to calm down. I went on to work with Angel a total of ten times, with each session lasting about an hour in length.

I learned a lot from working with Angel, such as how important it was to calmly negotiate and respect her feelings and alpha position at the National Eagle Center. I also learned that my honesty and sincerity of intention to help her could prevail and that fear prevents the encounter of healing from taking place. I have encountered all kinds of different fears in my encounters with various species of both tame and wild animals.

It appears that my intention to be of service is a key ingredient for a successful Rolfing session. Curiosity about finding a way for this body, with its accumulated injuries and traumas, can be positively affected by my experience, skills and intuition, seems to also be of primary importance.

MaryBeth Garrigan gives an update two years later on Harriet, Angel, Donald and Columbia. Spring 2009

Getting blood flow is a lot of what happens with feather growth, and the molt will indicate in their growth what the blood flow is like, how healthy the circulation system is, especially on the side that is affected by an injury.

Because of Harriet's injury, we have always been very cognizant of how she grows those new feathers in, especially on her left side where she has had an amputation and feather follicle damage, because many times those feathers will grow in crooked; the feathers will bend as they grow and point out. That can be problematic in that when she hits a perch wrong inevitably a blood feather, which has blood in it while it's growing, will break and there will be some bleeding. We have to be careful to make sure that the bleeding coagulates because if it doesn't, a bird could literally bleed to death if the feather shaft is large enough.

When she does break a blood feather, we have to put her in a little crate just to keep her quiet until that feather coagulates. We watch for when the bleeding has stopped before we put her back out. This year I can only think of one instance where we had to put her into the crate where normally it would have been several times over the year. She has done a lot of traveling this year, going full bore, and not having much of a problem.

She seems healthier than I've seen her in previous years, and I think that she has been sitting better. She hasn't been Rolfed in about five months, and it's amazing that during the two years that Briah has been seeing her—since May of 2007—this is the first time that she has had a problem.

She had something happen with her toe this week that may have started as a piercing underneath, like a hangnail that blew up into an infection, and she was hitting her perches crooked because I think it was sore. We have taken care of the infection at the Raptor Center, and that seems improved with the medication. We have been cleaning out the little infected area and now the swelling is down and I think she is sitting a little better.

There were times when she might be a bit agitated for five to ten minutes and try to bite at me but would settle right into the work as soon as I had my hands on her. I went on to work with Angel a total of ten times, with each session lasting about an hour.

With today's Rolfing session, I observed Harriet putting more weight back on that foot. I could feel again the vascularization in that foot because the foot is hot. It gets warm during the work and I think that helps with the healing process. It starts moving some of that infection out by bringing in new blood flow with its healing elements and nutrients. So she is standing solidly on both feet again.

While I hold her on the perch during a session, she sometimes starts feeling heavy on the glove. It's like she just sinks into my glove, and normally she sits pretty lightly. Today I felt this heaviness, a grounding of my feet into the floor that was very heavy and solid, like there was transference of some kind right through me and into the ground. I have felt that in my arm before, but today I felt it all through my body and into my feet. That was pretty amazing. I think of it as the connection that bird handlers have with the birds at some level.

It didn't take her long to get back in the saddle with the Rolfing work. She just seemed to say, "Okay, it's Briah." It just took about thirty seconds. I think that she will benefit from the session today and get back on track again after the foot injury. Now that she is starting her molt again it is good to get that alignment back.

Harriet is twenty-eight years old now and her health has been outstanding. She has been great with all the traveling and the way she's been uti-

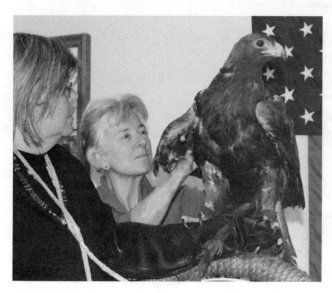

My first experience Rolfing Donald, a golden eagle.

lized at the Center. She has traveled around the state of Minnesota. She has been to sun dances out in South Dakota. She has been to New York, Washington, and Congress. She was on the Colbert Show in June, 2007, and I felt like Harriet was calmer than I was. There were cameras, lights, and lots of production people around, and Harriet was as calm as could be, centered, and solid. She has had a delegation from China with us, and people from all over the world have come up the Mississippi to see the eagles and the Eagle Center. She does well, and that's a twenty-eight-year-old bird. We're hoping we can keep her going until she's in her forties.

In the wild, an eagle is lucky to live until they are twenty years old, and most eagles die by twenty or twenty-five. There have been a few reports of a twenty-nine-year-old eagle, and perhaps a thirty-year-old eagle, which is very rare in the wild. Harriet was injured when she was about nineteen, and that's about when you might expect that to happen. Eagles start to move arthritically at nineteen and then they sometimes succumb to the pressures of trying to survive in the wild. In Harriet's case, and I say this ironically, "luckily" she was hit by a vehicle. If we look at it in that sense, she would have died of starvation or some other thing, and now she is an ambassador, and she has free health care benefits (laughs). She's got great insurance! She has great food, and I think she is thriving.

Donald, our golden eagle, had a right wing injury. He has been Rolfed about four times over the last eight months. He has adapted very well to the Eagle Center and we have to get Briah back with him. Since Briah was last here, his right side feathers have shown a different fraying pattern than on the left side. Since his molt he has been fraying up again. This tells me he's having some perching issues. We have been working on a couple of things so it will be interesting to see if we get him back on a schedule, if the Rolfing work can bring some improvement.

We have had to actually toughen Donald's feet rather than soften them.

With bald eagles their feet have to be flexible and kind of oiled to keep them from cracking, whereas with the golden eagles they need their feet toughened because they are a bird of the prairie and their feet aren't used in their natural way here. We have to put different ointments on his feet than we do the bald eagles. This is new for him, and he seems to be doing well in that respect. Now we're working on his balance issue, landing issues, getting him comfortable again. He is coming along. A lot of the staff work with him regularly on programs here, and getting adapted is always the hardest part for an eagle in its first year here. Things always happen.

Briah was able to Rolf Donald when he'd only been here a couple of months, and he's coming along fast. The first year is always the toughest because those birds tend to internalize stress and they blow up in different ways—like foot or feather growth problems. Donald has been having balance issues lately, so I think the Rolfing process will be a great benefit for him.

Angel is another bald eagle. Nothing stands in this bird's way. She is ferocious. She is the Furies. She is just amazing.

Eagles have an alpha role, but they don't have a pack. I think Angel's story is that she was around humans from a very early age. She was just a fledgling when they found her, and she is stuck in, "I am dominant female teenager" diva mode because she has never been beaten by another eagle. Usually when a young eagle is strutting her stuff, an older eagle will come and knock it off the perch or chase it out of the territory, and bring that eagle down a peg or two. Angel has not had that done, so she just thinks, "Well, that's just me, I'm just who I am!"

With Angel, we have to show her that we're not afraid of her. We have to face her with self assuredness and be strong in our sense of poise. She will take advantage of timidity: she hisses and tries to bite, and then bites harder the next time if the handler pulls away.

Angel has probably had around eight or ten sessions of Rolfing over the last year and a half. I notice that her

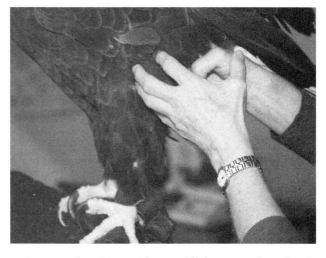

A close up of working with Donald's leg. Note the talons!

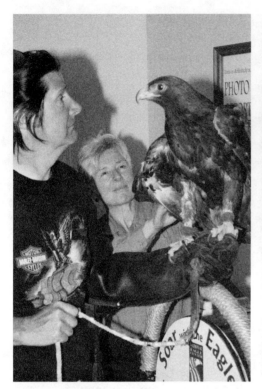
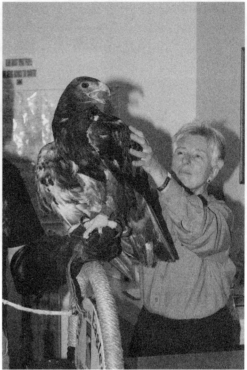

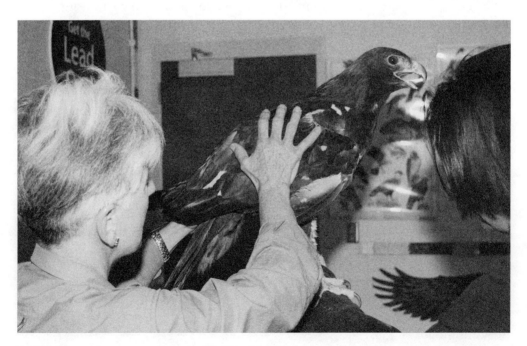

Establishing a deeper connection with Donald while eagle handler, Dennis Flint, assists.

feather tone has been really good. She has had really strong, balanced feathers, and little feather damage. I have not seen any cracked or broken feathers. She is in good condition with perfect wings and tail.

Columbia is a bald eagle who has been Rolfed about four times and she's in similar good condition: her feathers are looking really good. She had blood poisoning as a young bird so she has a learning disability. It has taken her longer to figure things out and she has a lot of anxiety. Her anxiety has lessened as the staff has worked with her—getting her out and giving her positive reinforcement. The Rolfing process has been helping her expand her limitations and paring down the anxiety. Eagles are not a touchy-feely kind of bird but with that special Rolfing contact they become less anxious about being touched. People often come close to them, and Columbia tends to become anxious when a lot of people closely surround her. After the Rolfing work, Columbia was more centered and could relax a little bit. She is coping with anxiety better.

All of the eagles have different personalities and different needs, but consistently, the response to receiving Rolfing sessions has been very positive. This last year has been just fabulous for them.

They have all had very few foot problems, even Donald during his first year, when we always expect these problems to happen. Harriet's toe infection is the first foot problem with her, but it is a minor thing.

Like humans, eagles can get respiratory infections; they can develop a fungal lung problem called aspergillosis. If their immune system becomes compromised, just like a cancer patient, they are vulnerable to aspergillosis, just as humans are. The fungal spores float in the air and when the immune system is compromised those fungal spores take over the respiratory system. With birds, that's the kind of thing that gets them more than a cold or even a bird flu. Traveling puts a lot of stress on their immune systems and we need to be careful about this fungus, so keeping them healthy and eating well is very im-

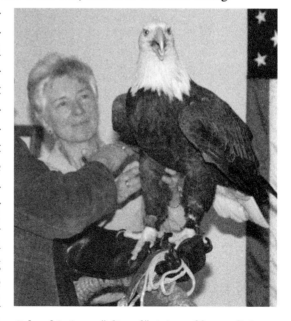

Columbia in an "altered" state, softly vocalizing as I work deeply into her leg.

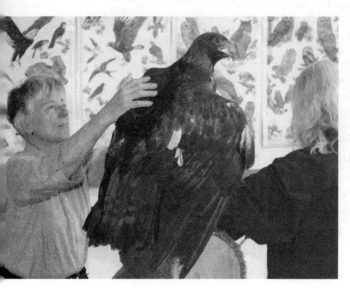

Donald in full regalia loving the work as eagle handler, Dottie Flint, assists me.

portant. They're doing very well and the Rolfing process has really helped them stay healthy.

Most of the staff at the Eagle Center have been really excited about the birds getting Rolfed. I think that the alternative medicine aspect of maintenance with birds is catching on. I thought it was very interesting that the Raptor Center at the University of Minnesota is doing acupuncture on birds now. We are obviously not a medical center in terms of clinical practice here, we are focused on education, but we like to try things that help to better the maintenance of our education birds and their quality of life.

Quality of life involves the little things that we think add to the birds' program and enrichment. Birds need enrichment in their lives when they don't have the wild. They need relationships or at least connections to their handlers in a different way than a bird in the wild would, and this is just another way of enriching their existence.

We take them out to the beach and let them go swimming in the river on Tuesdays (that's called beach day here). When the weather gets a little nice usually I will get a chance to get outside and get some sun and Vitamin D, and the birds do a little fishing! Harriet actually catches some fish. We try to do things that give the bird more stimulation and enjoyment. We actually engage them and they have little things that they do, little jobs, and it adds to their quality of life. Rolfing became a part of that.

Briah told me of a principle in Rolfing that it is through balance that you gain strength. I know that muscles can be built physically through nutrition and through manipulation. Raptors have very strong flight muscles that connect to the sternum and the wing, and when they atrophy through being injured like with Harriet, the muscles become very thin on one side and the sternum can be felt through the muscle. With enough work these muscles can be brought back into balance and that could probably be measured to some degree. With their weight gain, too, they will put on muscle tissue and lose muscle tissue, and you can measure a bird's health by what they call their keel. That is a measurable result.

Through the Rolfing process, Harriet appears to have more wingspan, and part of it might be from feeling better and getting more circulation to certain joints, so she has been able to extend more. That again helps with balance because, just like a tightrope walker when they hold out their arms on a tightrope, the birds use their wings for balance and landing. So for a bird it's important to be able to have extension, to be able to perch right and to feel good.

After Harriet's foot and wing incident she has not been able to land well on her perches for the last couple of months. It shows how one little thing can snowball and throw off the whole thing. Birds are like ice skaters—their perching balance is literally on the skate blade so to the extent that they're Rolfed and aligned, it makes their skating entirely different. We'll just have to keep working on it!

Feeling the benefits from a number of Rolfing® SI sessions Harriet now has the ability to completely open and spread her wings. With Scott Mehus, Education Coordinator, assisting and Bridget Beforg, Program Specialist, looking on in amazement.

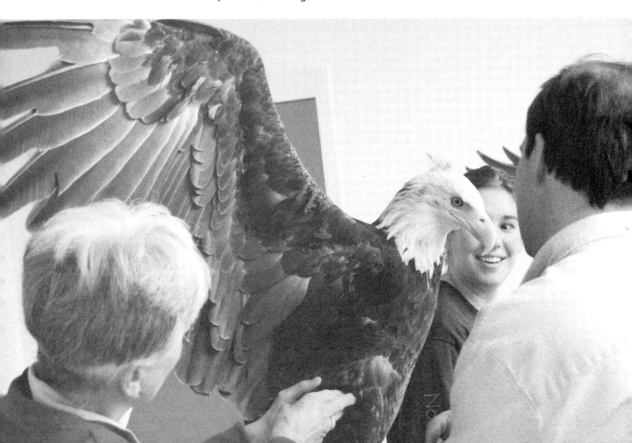

Too Afraid To Be Herself

Cindy Davis, on her dog, Gracie

Gracie is an Australian Shepherd who is about three and a half years old. I brought her in for Rolfing® sessions with Briah because she was having some behavioral difficulties. She was a very fearful dog—fearful of everything, such as people coming to the door. She would bark at them incessantly whether they were known to her or not, and she would react aggressively. We tried to train her (or I tried to train myself to train her) but we got nowhere. She's a pretty smart and strong-willed dog. She would get aggressive with me and my partner, Cathy, if we put our faces near hers when she didn't want that. She has bitten us a couple of times and that's where the behaviorist came in, and the Rolfing® came in later.

Working With the Fear Response

We hired an animal behaviorist from the University of Minnesota about nine months ago. She made a home visit and assessment, then suggested a way to try to train Gracie to obey us. We were to start with training her to not bark at the door when someone knocked.

We had determined that the biting was situational and unpredictable—that if she didn't want me to put my face in her face, then she would bite. She is actually a loving dog and wants to give kisses when she feels like it. So we just stopped putting our faces next to hers and avoided the situation altogether. A lot of vets recommend putting a dog down once they've bitten their owner, but we just didn't think her behavior called for that extreme a solution.

I had been through the Rolfing process myself and I told Briah about

Gracie's problem. A lot of the reason that I was attracted to coming to see Briah was the wide range of individuals she works on, her great expertise, and especially her work with animals. That suggested something to me about her.

When I had completed my Rolfing series with Briah I decided to bring Gracie in for Rolfing. Clearly, Briah had straightened me out, so to speak. My chest opened up and I am able to breathe fully now. When I first came in I had a lot of aches and pains everywhere—in my hips, shoulders, neck, joints, and knees. When I stood, Briah showed me that I had this leaning thing going on which I was unaware of. It affected everything about me. Being more physically balanced now, I've lost some of those chronic pains: I was unable to raise my left arm all the way because it would catch and get this nerve-like pain. That has gone away and having my body be more in balance and less in pain makes me a happier person.

My energy level has been pretty consistent since the Rolfing, and I think I'm more stable emotionally since I've started taking care of my body. After the positive results I had, taking Gracie in for Rolfing seemed like a good step. As of this writing, Gracie is getting her fourth session from Briah.

When I took Gracie in for her first session she did not want to be there. She kept trying to go back to the car and was very apprehensive. We had to coax her to even sit down so Briah could start working on her.

We did the first session outside so there were distractions like squirrels and people walking by, and I really had to hold her. Briah worked toward her back area which seemed to be causing Gracie problems and I was afraid that she might bite Briah. She had a lot of tightness back there. She was pretty strong-willed about where you touched her, or if you tried to do anything with her for that matter. She was very apprehensive and that's usually when the biting behavior would happen. By the end of that first session though, she was relaxed and not afraid of Briah's manipulations.

In the week after that first session she looked more relaxed in her physical appearance. It was like she'd stretched out or something. She looked puffier. She looked like she had lost weight, or was in good physical shape. She was longer. I noticed when I looked at her from the side that she actually had a waist. She had always been a compact dog and the vet commented once that she didn't have a waist which made her look overweight. She actually weighs about the same as she always has, but it's distributed more evenly now.

The next session was about a week or two later and she was very excited to come to Briah's. She ran to the door. So she has come to enjoy it, I think, or look forward to it. She loves to see Briah. Her tail goes around in a helicopter fashion which is what she does when she's happy to see someone.

Losing Fear

Something interesting happened after a couple of sessions—something we didn't expect. One of her chronic fears was to loud noises like thunder. She would be terrified and try to get under anything. The bathroom seemed especially safe to her, behind the toilet. She was just so afraid, and there was no comforting her. She would pant and shake, and try to escape. She was utterly terrified and could not be consoled. We would try to get her to come close so we could pet her, but petting her and talk-

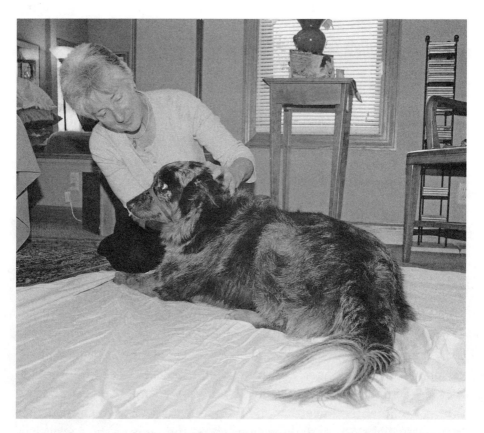

Gracie, a three-and-a-half-year-old Australian shepherd who used Rolfing® SI to go from fear and aggression to confidence and calm.

ing to her just did no good. She didn't want to sit by us, she just wanted to go where she felt it was safest. Watching that was sad for all of us because, you know, what could we do? It's the weather!

Without knowing that it would happen, the Rolfing actually helped her with that. She isn't afraid of thunderstorms anymore and that fear went away after that second or third session. It was a total shock.

We've had some pretty bad thunderstorms here lately in the middle of the night, many of them in the last two weeks. She has a little bed that she sleeps in at the foot of our bed. Before, during a thunderstorm she would not stay in her bed, it was "get me out of here!" But just the other night there was a thunderstorm and she slept through it! This happened after her third session—that's when we really noticed the change and made the connection. That has to be it, because that's really the only thing that's changed in her life.

Another thing that's happened is that she enjoys sitting with the front door open, which we never let her do before because she was such a barky dog. We have a storm door with a lot of glass in it, and now she likes to sit in front of that and watch people walk by—people with dogs, too. Not all dogs, she will go crazy at some of them and there's an Elkhound that she still hates. But for the most part, she sits there totally relaxed, watching—it's amazing. So she has settled down.

The accumulated affects of those three sessions has made a big difference. We're still hoping that her barking behavior when people come to the door will stop. I don't know if this last session will make that happen or not.

True Nature Emerges

There haven't been any more issues with her biting at anyone, but we don't put ourselves in that position with her either. She just seems a little more relaxed and looks a little more trusting. She now barks in excitement when people she knows come over. With strangers there's a different thing going on; it's definitely an aggressive bark and protective—not just a greeting bark—which is probably part of the nature of her breed.

She is generally more calm and much less anxious. Before Rolfing, when Cathy came home Gracie would bark in happiness to see Cathy, and now she is calm. She comes up and wags her tail and waits for the pets that will come. She seems to have a lot less anxiety.

Briah observed that Gracie has really nice movement through her whole body now and looks long. When she's off the leash and running I notice that she is longer and her strides are longer. I don't know if it's possible but she seems like she enjoys it more.

She has become really fond of chasing a stick and trying to get it on one bounce. She's playful and yet serious about it at the same time, which is more true to her breed. She seems more athletic. She likes going after the stick because she's a herding dog and so she'll bark at the stick as she is running toward it and circling around it. She reminds me of an athlete more so than before. She likes taking sharp corners and playing. Briah had remarked about her hind end being tied up, and her not being capable of that kind of quick movement and jumping and leaping without it causing her some distress.

I notice the instincts of her breed coming out more, like her innate potential has surfaced or been unleashed. I see that instinct show up in her playing with the stick and sometimes when a service person comes to our house. If they seem apprehensive of her she might nip at their heels just to keep them in line. This isn't such a good idea, of course, so I leave her behind a closed door usually. But it's part of her herding behavior, and watching her take on her true nature has been one of the welcome benefits of the Rolfing.

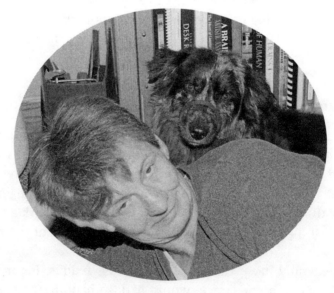

Gracie, with her owner Cindy.

Bringing out the Essence of an Animal

Carol Peterson, on her dog, Shelby Morgan

I had been going to Dr. Mary Rutherford at Crescenterra Health Center for many years and she finally got to a point where she felt she could not do anything more for me, and I was referred to Briah for Rolfing®. I hadn't ever heard about Rolfing so I was a little hesitant. Mary said that it would work well for me if I could combine the Rolfing and her chiropractic treatments. It was eight years ago that I met Briah.

I had fourteen sessions of Rolfing and during those sessions I started talking about dogs. I had lost my dog and was thinking about getting another. Briah had a golden retriever by the name of Shelby at the time, and she brought her dog to some of the sessions. She knew the grief I was feeling and it was very kind and caring of her to bring Shelby. During that Rolfing process I eventually got my golden retriever and Briah said, "You know, your puppy would benefit greatly from Rolfing." I was not aware of the animal Rolfing until she mentioned it.

I named my puppy after Briah's dog, Shelby. Actually, she is called Shelby Morgan because I also named her after Mary Rutherford's daughter, Morgan. I love the two names and I couldn't decide which name I wanted so I combined them. She is Shelby Morgan Peterson. The name has a soft spot for me because Briah lost her dog who was just a love, really a sweet dog.

Shelby was a gift to me from my husband, Mike, for Valentine's Day. She was about ten weeks old when we got her from the kennel. Briah had explained to me that as beneficial as Rolfing had been to me as a human, it was more beneficial to newborns, whether they are a human infant or an animal infant, because they are all bound up in the birth canal. The litter may be as large as nine puppies and Shelby may have been at the bottom of the pile getting twisted and turned. She said Shelby would benefit for the rest of her life by getting organized both emotionally and physically early on. She would become very agile and everything about her would be improved with Rolfing. So I thought, why not? She deserves every opportunity.

Rolfing SI for the Puppy

I was a little worried about coming in with a little rambunctious puppy—you know how puppies are! I brought her into the treatment room and she had never seen Briah before. Shelby was just doing her thing; Briah had a ball for her and she was moving around quite a bit as Briah worked on her with the deep penetration of her hands. There is almost a spiritual side to Briah when she Rolfs. I was amazed to see her affect on this hyper puppy. Shelby went from active sitting to lying down, and then her head actually draped over the side of the table and she just slept throughout the session.

Shelby had two sessions, and from then on I saw a difference in her spirit and her movement that has lasted until this very day. She is more

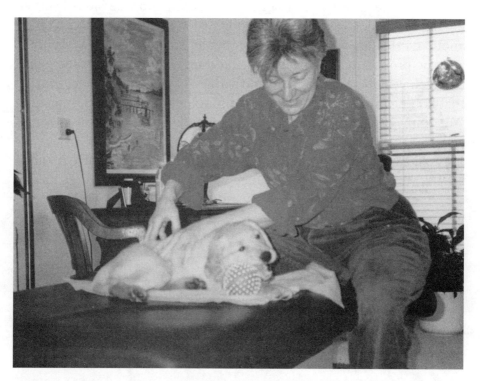

Shelby Morgan, a golden retriever under three months old off to a good start with Rolfing® SI.

agile, and I think she is a happy dog. Every time Mike and I have some-one here who has never seen Shelby, that is the first thing they say, "Gee, she's a happy dog." She's seven-and-a-half years old now, and her move-ments are still those of a younger dog, which I think is because we had her Rolfed as a puppy. Briah explains it as uncluttering the dog's life, both physically and emotionally, and it allows a puppy to grow into who they should be. I was just really impressed with that.

Overcoming Injury

Shelby started having a mysterious problem later in her adult life. She became unable to get off the floor easily and we worried that it might be an aging problem like arthritis or hip dysplasia. Before I took her to the vet I called Briah for her opinion. She had us bring her over, and I was impressed to see how Shelby still recognized Briah, many years later. She became very calm. It was that spiritual thing that I had seen before. The love that Briah has for animals that's in her heart and her hands—it projects out of her hands and into the animals.

She did the session outdoors which she thought might be more com-fortable for Shelby. It was a beautiful summer day and she spread a blan-ket out on the ground, knelt down alongside Shelby and proceeded to Rolf her right there. Because it was such a beautiful day I think it was just enjoyable for all of us in that natural setting.

This was before I took Shelby to the vet and we didn't know that she had a torn cruciate ligament. I suspect this pre-surgery Rolfing helped her recover more quickly from the surgery later. That day it was easy to see that the Rolfing took away the pain and helped her relax. Briah touched Shelby as if she knew exactly where to go with the placement of her hands, and not just in her leg where the problems were, but in dif-ferent areas. Shelby just lay her head down and accepted the help. She looked back at Briah several times and she licked her hand, which Briah and I both commented on. It seemed like she was saying thank you.

Shelby had three sessions of Rolfing and then I took her to the univer-sity vet hospital for X-rays. It was then that we discovered the torn cruci-ate ligament and Shelby had surgery. I think her recovery from surgery was faster than normal because of the Rolfing. I mentioned it to her vet, Dr. Anderson, who wasn't as familiar with Rolfing as we were, but still he said it certainly couldn't have hurt, and that she showed signs of a really good recovery. We picked her up the day after her surgery and she was straining on the leash and trying to walk as best she could. I couldn't believe how resilient she was.

Finding Essence

I have heard Briah say that one of the purposes of Rolfing for humans or animals is to bring out the essence of that being. When people say about Shelby, "She seems like such a happy dog," that's it right there. Mike noticed it as well. He was skeptical about Rolfing at first. He always needed to be convinced of anything alternative like acupuncture or Rolfing. But he is the one who noticed that Shelby became so limber and agile that she could lie with her legs out in the back. He became truly impressed when she started to roll and kick her feet up. Those were visual signs that this treatment really did do something and he has been all for it ever since. He might even get Rolfed now himself, and I don't think he would have considered it before this. When you see your animal respond to Rolfing and watch it bring out the essential nature of your pet, you can't help but be impressed.

Shelby began life as the runt of the litter. She seemed to have a defiant streak in her so she was not an easy puppy. She was very hard to housebreak. She would chew on things and ruin them deliberately. She never listened and I couldn't correct her. It was not easy to do anything with her. After her two Rolfing sessions her personality started changing; she was easier to direct, less defiant. She was not as hyper and did less chewing. Puppies are hyper by nature, but she was out of control. I was so impressed and amazed at how even-keeled she became that I talked about it for months!

Her essence is to be a very high-spirited, independent, happy dog that loves to play. She's become very loving and well-adjusted. The word "organized" has stayed with me as a good description of

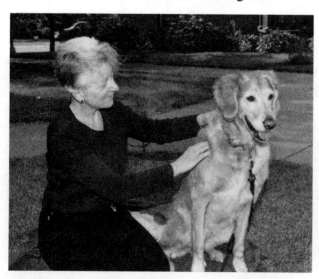

Shelby Morgan, at ease and at peace, receiving a Rolfing® SI session from me seven-and-a-half years later.

what happens. Shelby became more organized in her life. But it wasn't just organized physically—I had the feeling that she came into *herself* more, and the phrase "bringing out your essence" made sense to me.

Her movements are very good, even now, years later. She is not suffering from any of the problems that often show up years after surgeries—like neck problems or the other leg gets injured. Vets say there is a 50 percent chance of later problems. But Shelby has stayed healthy and mobile and I'm sure it's because of Briah and how she does the Rolfing.

The Animal Response to Rolfing SI

One of the things that I was amazed to watch as Shelby got Rolfed was the total lack of resistance she had. This puppy started the session sitting upright and suddenly she was laying down with her head actually hanging over the side of the table—completely OUT. She simply surrendered to Briah. The dog was totally cooperative during Briah's manipulations. She was at ease and at peace. I can imagine how Briah is with the other kinds of animals that she works with like eagles, and how babies would respond this way as well.

It looks like they are in an altered state. They do not seem to experience it as uncomfortable. Perhaps what they're experiencing is how deeply healing this kind of touch is. They can come to Briah in tremendous pain and allow her to work deeply, and then incorporate the work, or as Briah says, integrate it.

Before Briah begins a session with either an animal or a human, she gets into this zone where she organizes her own energy around them. She is focusing just on them and it has a spiritual sense to it. It is a wonderful thing and I am impressed with her as a Rolfer™. It seems to be the perfect work for her. Maybe the Rolfing helped bring out her essence as well, and it is a genuine caring nature that she has.

I was very grateful to be introduced to Rolfing, both for what it has done for me emotionally and physically, and what it has done for Shelby. We pet owners want to do whatever it takes for our pets to lead a healthy and happy life, just like parents do with their children. Rolfing is something Shelby and I will both go back to as we age because I am sure that we'll continue to benefit greatly.

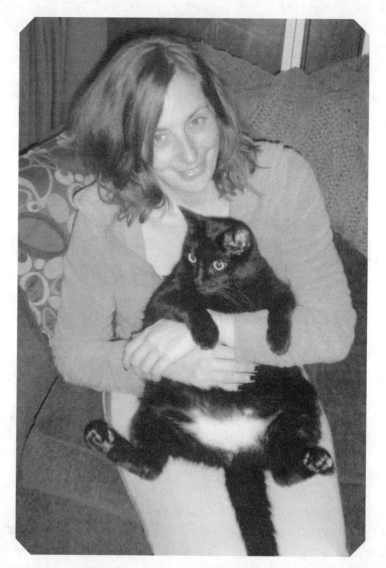

Haley and Texas: "Happy to have my sweet kitty back."

The Legend of Texas James

Haley Lasché writes about her cat, Texas James

When Texas James first came to me, he'd already lived with two of my friends for some time, and Texas and I had an affinity for each other. Whenever I attended parties at his home, he would sit on my lap and purr away until I got up to socialize. Then he would hide in the bathroom sink licking fresh water and enjoying the private attentions of party-goers. He was a bit shy but also curious. I loved how he would stare up at me with ocean green eyes trying to take in the idea of me. I loved how, when he was comfortable, he'd roll onto his back and expose the white heart of his tummy. When his mom came to me asking if I would take care of him, it wasn't a difficult decision. Though I had never lived with a cat before, I had always wanted one. I knew Texas and I could have a great kitty-parent relationship. I was ready to welcome him into my home.

The first night Texas spent in my apartment was so much fun. I had used the previous two weeks to read cat books and prepare my home for him. I had read that cats feel comfortable in small rooms, so I set up my bathroom with blankets in my tub, food and water dishes in one corner and a small litter box in the other. On the drive from his old house to my apartment, he meowed the whole way. By the time we reached our destination, I was afraid his anxiety level would be high and his actions would be unpredictable. I brought him into the bathroom, opened the latch on his cat carrier and cracked the carrier's door open. I snuck out of the bathroom and left the door slightly ajar. A few minutes later, I peeked around the hallway corner to see a little green eye the size of a silver dollar peering out at me. As I opened the door wider, he scurried across the grey carpet and thoroughly sniffed every corner of the apartment. He explored every inch until he saw the most intriguing sight: himself reflected in my mirrored closet door. When I fell asleep that night, he was staring mesmerized by his own eyes. When I woke the next morning, he was lying down, nose just inches from the same mirror. He must have always known he was a handsome cat but finally, he had found the proof of it.

He was shy of my friends (especially those with whom he had lived). He would hide in my bathroom or under the sofa. His former moms would tell stories of how he was weaned too early, how they would wake in the middle of the night with his black velvet frame lying long against them as he suckled the skin on their necks. He had separation anxiety, and while his posture was strong, each of his reactions carried at least a small insecurity behind it. Some insecurities were larger than others. When the chimes on the front door would "ching," Texas would run for one of his hiding spots. He would stay there through meals and movies, peeking out only when he felt certain no one would take him away. Once he began to feel comfortable, he would pass against my visitors' legs, arms, backs and faces (when he could reach them). He would come back and forth against them so many times he eventually earned the nickname, "Drive-by-Kitty."

Texas and I moved into one new apartment, then another. For each new move, I would put a pile of dirty clothes on the floor of my bedroom closet. He would run for that nest and curl into a ball, his silver dollar eyes blinking open at gradually smaller radii with each day we passed in our new home. I would pet his head and tell him, "You're staying with me." He would respond with a low and raspy purr. After a series of days, I would come home from work to find him in the middle of living room rug, lying on his back with his legs stretched long, white heart belly signaling that X marks the spot of home.

After a time, a "foster" cat (Todd) came to live with us. Todd had been another friend's cat and had spent weekends with us before he moved in. The two cats would get crazed on catnip and wrestle each other. Their wrestling matches always ended with bites turned to licks turned to naps. Texas was the big brother, the one who always managed to get control over the warm spot on the sofa, the best view out the window and the first pick in the food bowl. Over the course of a few years, Texas gained a little weight, and it was impossible to get him to exercise. Whenever anyone would try to play with him, he would roll over on his back and stretch his white-hearted belly long. Wrestling with Todd (in that same posture) was the only kind of play he could be coerced into. Todd would jump out at him from behind the sofa, run a circle around Texas, crouch (wiggling his backside) and pounce on him. Texas would lie there, waiting for contact, then kick Todd in the head repeatedly. He would stumble off when the blows became too much, but Todd always came back for more.

While Texas would never let Todd win, he still adored his little brother. One weekend, Todd somehow managed to find his way off our second story balcony, and when I returned, there was Texas standing on the precipice of the platform, meowing after what I can only assume was Todd's jumping off point. He was inconsolable for a week until we found Todd. When Todd was finally returned to our home, Texas followed him everywhere for three days, until Todd asserted (in his kitty way) that he had a need for some privacy.

Texas loved to be held. He would jump on my chest and curl into a cat with no legs. I would pet him with long strokes from ears to tail. He would purr (and sometimes drool). He'd snuggle that way until he had too much; then, he would roll over on his side and let me hold him like a baby until he fell asleep. Some nights he would sleep on my feet, but more often, he would sleep in one spot and position on the sofa. In the morning, he would stare at me as I got out of bed and washed my face. I would come over to his sofa, whisper "good morning, sweet kitty" and kiss his ears. He would purr softly and wait for me to fill the food dish before jumping off his resting place and starting his day. In the first several years that I had Texas, he seemed content to be loved, to be appreciated. He was happy to be with Todd and me. He would go from zero to purr in a matter of seconds.

In the summer of 2008, the three of us moved into a two-story house. In just a couple of weeks, both cats lost a few pounds (a result of chasing each other up and down the stairs). Texas discovered the greatest joy of living in a house: lying in the windows and watching the bird feeders and all the creatures that frequented them. Everything seemed happy in the house, but over the course of those years, Texas began to get lazy. He was having a hard time reaching all the parts of his fur to clean himself. He was getting fatter and fatter. His patience for playing with Todd began to wane; he would fight for a few seconds, then just lie there and let Todd lick him. When Todd would try to clean Texas's hind-quarters, Texas would swat at him and run away. His hind-quarters were getting more and more unkempt, and without help from Todd, I began to pick up the slack. Texas would whine and hiss while I cleaned his backside; however, it was no incentive to take matters into his own paws. In fact, he started caring less and less about his hygiene the more I helped.

In the months before I took Texas for Rolfing® SI, he would commit to washing only his front paws and face. His fur was matting down on both sides of his haunches. It was so thick I would have to cut the knots out with a scissors. I bought a variety of cat brushes and cleaned up his posterior whenever it was messy. Texas was embarrassed by both of those activities. He didn't want me to clean him and he was even more resistant if Todd was around. He would whine like a sad dog and plead at me with his green eyes. But I wanted him to be healthy and cared for. I would thank him for his patience with catnip, treats and scratches to his ears, yet he didn't react in the Pavlovian way I'd hoped he would. His messiness continued.

In July of 2010, I had an opportunity to travel for three weeks. I found a cat sitter who had pets of her own, but who lived close enough to come by and spend some time with my boys each day. While I know Texas and Todd loved their cat sitter (both before and after she came to sit with them), when I returned from my travels, there was something very different about them. First, Todd had an insatiable urge to go outside. Second, Texas had gained a significant amount of weight and would nip at anyone who petted him longer than he desired. His threshold for attention had become an unpredictable boundary; sometimes he couldn't get enough and sometimes he couldn't stand to be touched within a few seconds of sitting down on my lap. In the mornings, when I kissed his ears to wake him up, he ignored me. If I tried to linger a bit longer or pet him waiting for a purr, he would retreat to an upstairs room far away from me and his breakfast bowl.

If I was snuggling with Todd, his reactions were even worse. Texas had always been a little jealous when Todd co-opted the best spot in the house, but after my trip, he found Todd's presence unbearable. If Todd was sitting on my lap, Texas would sneak up and bite him, trying to pull him down off of me. If Todd was on the best pillow, Texas would bear hug and drag Todd off of the good spot with his front claws. If Texas wanted to be in a room where Todd was, he would chase him out. Just when I thought his jealousy couldn't get worse, it began to resemble shame. Not only did Texas want to keep Todd from being loved, if Todd witnessed Texas receiving affection, Texas had to escape. He would jump from whoever was holding him, pushing off extra hard with his back feet, and sometimes scratching until he broke skin. And if Todd dared entered the room Texas was in, Texas would scurry off for a private place. He would barely let me look at him, but Todd, the cat he once treated like a little brother, had turned into an enemy so terrible that Texas couldn't even breathe the same air as he did.

A few weeks after my return, a stray cat adopted our house. She was declawed in the front and Todd would cry every time she came to one of the doors (so, of course, we named her Jolene). Todd was an alarm that sounded whenever she came near; he was hungry for a cat friend who wouldn't reject him. Texas, on the other hand, took her arrival as an attack. When she came to our yard, he would follow her from window to window without blinking. His eyes captured every possible misstep, and his behaviors against Todd became even more extreme. He began pushing him around, waking him during naps and biting his throat when they were wrestling.

Their style of play, once lighthearted and loving, had turned dangerous. On one incredibly scary evening, Texas chased Todd past Todd's "I've had enough" hiss, even past Todd's attempt to hide in a cardboard box on the floor. Texas chased him out of the box and shouldered him up against the side of a table where he put Todd in a kitty version of a half Nelson and tried to use his powerful jaws to break Todd's neck. After breaking up the fight and trying to keep them both calm for the night, I tried to deal with Texas's anger. I put Soft Paws on his front toe nails so that the tearing of skin could be minimized. I bought him a mouse toy covered in rabbit fur so he could lick it and pretend it was prey. I even bought him a raw hide to keep him from using Todd as a chew toy.

He stopped eating the second anyone came into the kitchen. He would scurry away as if he had been caught doing something naughty. Though I rarely saw him eat, he continued to gain weight, and when he was walking on the wooden floors on the second floor of the house, it sounded like a six-foot-tall man had invaded.

I tried changing his diet so that only half of what he ate was kibble and the other half was organic canned food. Texas was resistant. He waited for Todd to eat up all of the canned food and then scarfed down as much as he could of the kibble. I finally found a flavor that he liked, but he still wouldn't eat the food. He'd only lick the top until he'd had enough of the flavor.

The night that Briah came to work on Texas was the biggest shift. He was calm for the first few minutes, he whined for the next, he hissed for few minutes after and then we took a break. After the break he continued to go back and forth between whining and hissing, so we took a second break. During each break, Texas ran out of the room. However, a few minutes later, he let us know that he was ready for more Rolfing SI. He came back into the room, rubbed up against my legs and reminded us of the Drive-by Kitty he used to be. The next day, Texas was a different cat.

When I woke, I put on the coffee and opened the curtains in the living room. I kissed him on his head. "Good morning, sweet kitty," I said, and he responded with a purr. I had become so unaccustomed to his enjoyment of this simple act that I felt I had to test it a little longer. I stroked his ears and scratched his nose, but he only purred louder and lifted his chin for more scratching. I went to phase two: breakfast. As soon as I cracked open the can of turkey and salmon, Texas came scurrying into the kitchen. He sat in the place where I normally put his food dish and waited patiently for me to place the glass bowl under his nose. He ate about half of what I had given him before strolling off to clean his whiskers. The bath got so far as his back legs before he moved on to one of his favorite spots in the window. I couldn't believe what I was seeing. Texas, who had given up baths completely, was showing off his limber cat nature. He was stretching, and that's when it occurred to me that maybe what I had been assuming was laziness was really the result of a structural issue.

He was stretching, and that's when it occurred to me that maybe what I had been assuming was laziness was really the result of a structural issue. I had thought his change in behavior was completely emotional. It never occurred to me that my big, black, loveable cat had been physically suffering.

I had thought his change in behavior was completely emotional. It never occurred to me that my big, black, loveable cat had been physically suffering.

Within three days, Texas was a cleaning machine. He began to lick the midsection of his tail and his back legs more and more frequently. Soon, the patches of fur that I'd had cut off of him began to grow back. He was walking with a lighter step. He would sneak up on me while I was reading. I wouldn't even know he was there until he let out a tiny 'meow', a request to sit on my lap and be loved.

Then, about a week after his first session I saw Texas do something I never knew he could do. He was sitting on the living room table watching the finches fight over seed when he noticed that I was sitting on the sofa two feet away from him. He walked to the edge of the table, prepped and leapt onto the arm of the sofa. He hopped right down onto the seat, putting his front paws on my lap and starting to purr. My poor Texas, the cat who in the last several months could stand neither physical activity nor snuggles was instigating both in a matter of seconds. All of the traumas he had experienced had disappeared, he was acting three years younger, and I was happy to have my sweet kitty back.

I had forgotten how he used to lie on my chest and purr, how he'd roll over on his side and let me hold him like a baby until he fell asleep. I had forgotten how he used to let me pet him until he would drool from the stimulation. He began to enjoy his food, and he reacted to the opening of the can like the "unzip" sound of his treats and catnip bags.

I wondered how long his contentment would last until one November day. I was watching the news and folding laundry. Texas was sleeping on the sofa next to me even though the volume on the TV was loud. Todd had jumped up to lick Texas's ears: a clear signal that it was time to play or at the very least fight for the warm spot. I assumed Todd would be kicked off the sofa in a few quick seconds. I continued folding and only half waited to hear the thump of rejected cat feet. I didn't pay any more attention to it than that. I was so wrapped up in the election drama of the gubernatorial race that I didn't even notice it happen. But as I went to place a freshly folded pair of jeans on the "done pile," I saw Todd curled up next to Texas, a second book end that had gone missing and finally had been returned to its rightful place. Both little tummies rising and falling in faint purrs like a happy end to a happy day.

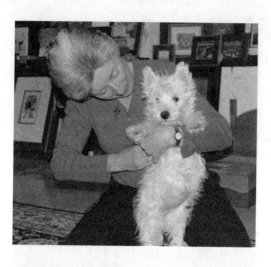
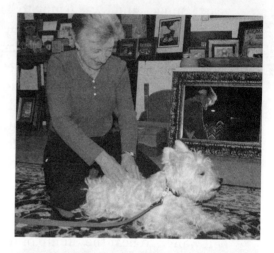
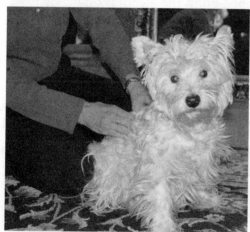
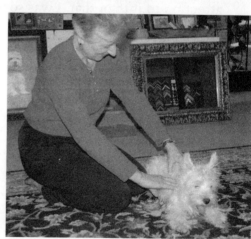

Brother and sister Stanley and Ann (West Highland terriers). Rolfing® SI helped transform them into harmonious and loving siblings.

Harmonizing the Pack:
From Competition to Companions

Cheryl Hoover, on her dogs, Stanley and Ann

Briah Anson was my customer at Captured Visions for six years. I had framed multiple pieces of art for her. I got a new puppy, a West Highland Terrier named Stanley. Stanley was the lucky recipient of several Rolfing® sessions with Briah.

When Briah would come into my framing shop she'd pet Stanley. She noticed that Stanley was extremely tight and compacted. This breed in general tends to be athletic, compacted, highly strung and tight. When we'd walk Stanley he'd constantly pull on his harness. Briah offered me the gift of some Rolfing for Stanley. She spent about an hour on two different occasions Rolfing him. Stanley only weighs seventeen pounds and most of it was extremely tight musculature. Briah knew that if he did not get some Rolfing now, that later in life he'd have some problems with his hind end.

After the first session I noticed that Stanley was more relaxed and agile. Before the session he was acting like a little old man at only two years old. He was somewhat lethargic and stiff and his gait had a little limp. He was obviously out of alignment which you could see when he walked down the street.

The second Rolfing session was a couple of months later. Stanley seemed very receptive to this. He greeted Briah with excitement as if he knew what was going to happen. He lay right down to allow Briah to get right to work on him. Again, Briah worked for close to an hour and Stanley was cooperative throughout. He would turn from side to side as if he was guiding the session. Occasionally he would lick Briah as if he was encouraging her to continue the session.

After this session Stanley ran around, full of energy and was wild, acting like a puppy. Something had been freed up in him. He seemed like a different dog. He even felt lighter. Both Briah and I noticed that his seventeen pounds seemed half the weight. He was playful, almost silly. He would engage me to play with him as he did when he was a puppy. After this second session he was also easier to walk. He was "lighter" on the leash and not such a struggle to walk.

Then we got Ann, another Westie, and everything changed. Ann was nine weeks old, and weighed three pounds when she came into our home. She was the most obnoxious girl any one of us had ever met, including Stanley. She was loud and demanding. She adored Stanley who wanted nothing to do with her. That continued for about five months. Ann was then spayed. The sassy loud demanding puppy turned into a pitiful baby who'd had surgery (with teeth removed the same day as the spaying). Briah came into the store that day without calling, which she'd always done. Briah wanted to see Ann. I was feeling protective and didn't want Briah to see her. Briah insisted on seeing her. Briah started on Ann with some energy work (Qi Gong). She gave her a homeopathic remedy, a dose of Arnica to help with the trauma of her surgery. Briah said this would reduce the inflammation from the surgery and the pain. I was still skeptical. Briah said I'd notice a change in Ann within an hour or two. In less than forty-five minutes we noticed a huge change in her. She started becoming playful, barking at Stanley, chasing him around. This was a huge difference in her behavior. By the next morning she was her regular self: loud, demanding, obnoxious—like nothing had happened.

Stanley was very upset with Ann and was uncharacteristically naughty. I asked Briah if she could work some magic on Stanley. The next day Briah came back to my store to work on Stanley. She gave Stanley a homeopathic remedy that would address his mental and emotional state. She also Rolfed him and gave him some hypnotic inductions regarding how important he is in our family and that he was still the "boy king" in the family. Briah says she's discovered that once an animal is in an altered state she can talk to them in such a way that they can understand it and as importantly, feel understood. From that day forward it was as if Briah had flipped a switch in Stanley's brain and he finally accepted Ann as a member of our pack. At that point I became a believer in Briah's work. It has been amazing to watch the dogs since Briah has worked on them.

Previous to the work, Ann would always want to snuggle with Stanley. He wanted no part of that. He'd growl at her to get away from him. After the Rolfing everything changed. He accepted Ann. He played with her in a gentle loving way. They now use each other as pillows and seem to comfort each other. It has been six months since the work has been completed and their relationship continues to be amazing to watch. Their bond is very strong. Stanley is protective of Ann. Their relationship is harmonious and they continue to play like loving siblings, to the point that they don't seem to need other dogs. If I hadn't seen it with my own eyes I don't know that I'd have believed the transformation. I tell everyone about the healing powers of Rolfing. I feel people's awareness needs to be raised regarding the power of Rolfing to heal our companion animals.

Expect the Unexpected:
Unleashing the Primal Animal

Interview with Carrie Voyles and Walker Mallory about their cats, Elwood and Rhiannon

Carrie Voyles: Elwood and Rhiannon are seven-year-old domestic shorthair cats. They're not siblings but we adopted them both at around six weeks, and they've lived together almost their whole lives. They were rescue cats. Elwood was found on a trail, he'd been abandoned or gotten lost and he was really freaked out. Rhiannon was adopted from a small shelter here in the Twin Cities.

They're both very sweet affectionate cats. Elwood is especially interested in people, loves to be around them, and is very, very socialized. Rhiannon is a little bit more aloof but still a pretty friendly and curious kitty. I was interested in getting Rolfing® sessions for them after hearing so many of Briah's stories about her work with pets.

They have a couple of behavioral issues that I was hoping would be helped. Elwood is really fixated on food and he's rather overweight because of that. I work at home and sometimes my husband does as well, so we're around a lot and he does pester us for food. I was hoping that the Rolfing sessions might calm down whatever anxiety it is that causes that, and help him feel a little more at ease emotionally. Rhiannon is a fairly well adjusted kitty, although she does have a little habit of tearing up paper. She mostly does that as a way of letting us know that she wants to eat; she'll find a piece of paper and just shred it into little bits.

Elwood has also had a couple of head injuries in his life. He had his head accidentally shut in a door as a kitten, and he also ran head-first into a window once, so both of those incidents may have given him little concussions. He had some apparent tender spots along his spine. When I would pet him or massage along his back, he would flinch a little or twitch in certain areas along his spine, so I know he probably had some muscular aches and pains or places where things weren't flowing fluidly. Being overweight may have exacerbated that for him too.

Rhiannon has been very athletic and can perform all kinds of feline feats, but Elwood is more grounded. He can jump four or five feet, but he doesn't get any more ambitious than that. He's pretty careful about jumping.

In the process of the Rolfing work, I was interested to see how they each responded differently during the sessions than I thought they would. With Elwood, who loves to be touched and cuddled, I thought he would just love it. With Rhiannon, who's not very much of a lap cat (she's very particular about whose lap and when and all that), I thought she would be a little more skittish with sitting still for an hour of Rolfing work—and it was just the opposite. These were long sessions—an hour and twenty minutes. Elwood had some periods during the sessions when he would really seem to settle in and get into some kind of deep space where he was receiving the work, but he had a bit of a hard time settling down into it the first half hour. Then he really got into it, and after that it was very smooth and it was easy for him to stay with it. He would occasionally get up, turn around, reposition himself. He didn't really want to leave, he was just antsy. He would even turn over on his back—Elwood loves to lie on his back anyway. It was a very relaxed and open position for him.

Rhiannon normally never lies on her back, but during the session I was amazed at how quickly she settled into receiving the work, and how much she wanted to spend time on her back so that Briah could work on her lower abdominal area, particularly around the psoas and all the hip muscles. She was very open and just incredibly receptive and relaxed. I almost never see her as relaxed as she was then. She's half Elwood's size; she weighs about nine pounds and Elwood is nineteen pounds. She was in my lap and Briah worked very deeply in this first session. Briah had met the cats several times before but they'd never interacted much—just-passing-by kind of greetings. But Rhiannon completely loved her Rolfing session.

A week later, Briah did second sessions with both cats, and this time Rhiannon responded the same, but Elwood couldn't settle down. He didn't get as deep into it as he did in the first session. Again, he didn't try to stop the session but he would stand up, turn around, flip over—he just seemed a little more restless.

I have seen behavioral changes in Elwood since we started the work, but they weren't what I anticipated. He hasn't calmed down with his obssession, rather he's switched his obsession from food (to some degree anyway, he still wants to eat a lot) to wanting to go outside. When he goes outside now he wants to hunt. We take them out on leashes because we live in a community where you are not allowed to let your cat out without a leash, they're not allowed to run free. We take them out usually once a day on leashes individually. Before their Rolfing sessions, Elwood just wanted to catch small bugs. He was never into chasing squirrels or chipmunks or any kind of little animal. He really was good at chasing bugs. He could detect where they were and he was very quick, he was good at it. He would eat them, so that was his big adventure, big enterprise. But since the Rolfing SI he wants to catch mammals! We have some voles that live here in the ground on a little hillside near our house and he'll see them from thirty feet away. He'll see one and march right up to where it is, then he will plop down on it and trap it. Soon it's jumping up trying to get away. He's carried one around in his mouth and tried to bring it inside to eat, but I wouldn't let him. I have never seen him display that type of true primal cat instinct for hunting.

Rhiannon, the female, is a hunter. She's caught things, and we don't like her to do that, but sometimes she's just so fast. Even on the leash she will catch a chipmunk and we make her let it go. But this is a first for Elwood. Seven years old, he's been outside on the leash every warm

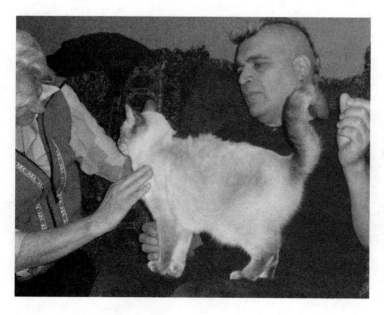

Rhiannon receiving Rolfing® SI as my Structural Integration colleague, Walker, looks on.

season since he has been a kitten, and he's never attempted to do this before, but now he is. It's pretty cool that he is rediscovering this part of himself. I have no idea why he didn't exhibit this behavior before; maybe he didn't feel as agile or his energy overall wasn't as high, and maybe he has more vitality now.

We did notice after the first session that when he sat his back line looked more smooth, it was longer and more curved, like there was more freedom of movement through his spine. He still likes to spend a lot of time on his back and I think that's partly because with his weight, that's a comfortable position for him, he can relieve some of the pressures that he feels from gravity that way. He still likes to eat about the same amount but he isn't quite as focused on that as his only source of plea-sure. He has other interests now like wanting to go out several times a day. He rarely gets to, we just don't have time, but he's asking for it. I'm not sure how that's going to work in the winter because there comes a time when he still wants to go outside but faced with the cold, he's like, "Aw no, this is too cold! We're not doing this!"

Walker Mallory: I see the most difference in Elwood. He's longer—not so hunched over like a raccoon. He's more catlike now. Upon awakening or as soon as he comes out to the kitchen in the morning, he's ready to go outside, and he's hunting out there. This afternoon there was a bird on this stop sign near the house, and Elwood stood there for quite a long

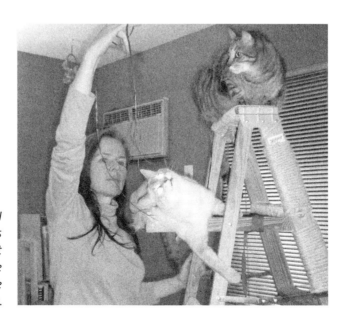

After the Rolfing® SI sesssion, Carrie enjoys the playful spirit of Rhiannon while Elwood, king of the mountain, looks on.

time, stalking the little bird. He's hunting and catching as well. He used to go out and just want to lie under a bush in the dirt, but now he walks around a lot more. He's been to the road with me a couple of times and out in the field quite a ways. He walked to the care facility nearby the other day, and he kept making noise, meowing and chittering. He likes walking on curbs, and there was a curb over there so I thought he just wanted on that curb. But I noticed about twelve feet before we got there that there is a bird feeder in front of the facility, and birds were everywhere. He was doing his little chittering noise, and as soon as I saw that that's what he was after, I picked him up and brought him over to a different curb. He seems to be expanding his territory.

CV: Elwood has always been really careful about controlling himself around nipping, but since the Rolfing work, he's not as careful. He's actually nipping more. He's more freely exercising that power that he knows he has to influence our behavior. We admonish and ignore him when he nips, but still, he persists. Maybe the sessions have awakened some need in him that has to do with jaw action or biting which might be progress for him, but it is an awkward stage in our household right now. He doesn't break the skin or nip out of meanness, but to get our attention and get what he wants, right now!

Briah Anson: It sounds to me like he's back in touch with some of his primal behaviors and is acting those out with both of you. He's been at one extreme with socialized behavior, having to be walked on a leash and so forth which cats don't naturally take to, and now he's bringing in this other end of the primal cat pole. I would expect that to balance out sometime.

CV: I think it will. I haven't noticed differences in Rhiannon's behavior other than for a few days after both sessions she and Elwood were very calm. It was like they'd spent a weekend at a meditation retreat. They weren't talking, they weren't pestering, they weren't interacting much. They were very serene and would sit and gaze for the rest of the evening after the session. The next day they continued to sit and gaze, and then they slept a lot. They obviously had a lot of integrating to do.

Rhiannon seems to be eating more than she had been and she is not as fussy about food. She was never underweight, but I feel a difference now when I touch her and palpate her muscles—she has a more filled out feeling. Not that she's fat, it's just that she feels more like an athlete's body feels. When you massage an athlete their tissue feels alive and firm yet plump, and activated. She feels more smoothly activated all over now. She had muscles before, but they were compacted and the bones were more promintent, and now I just feel this lovely muscle.

BA: I would describe it like the tissues felt very close to the bone before. There is one thing I wanted to mention because I had not experienced this with any of the cats that I've worked with. I distinctly remember during her first session, there were eight or nine times in that period of more than an hour where I felt this incredible energy or tingling sensation travel through my whole body. I understood that what I was putting out for Rhiannon was coming right back to me. It felt like she is this incredible little healer cat, and that really stayed with me. I remembered that you had described her as not quite as bright as Elwood because when you'd hide toys, she wouldn't know where you put them, or she didn't seem interested in those kind of games. I was amazed to feel this high level of healing energy coming back toward me. I started telling her, oh, you're just a little healer! And then I started getting these intense, and to me, meaningful, looks from her. I remember being very taken by that.

CV: She seems to have different perceptions or a different level of interaction with her environment than Elwood does. She's very interested in sitting on Walker, my husband. She pretty much wants to be on him, all the time. I have noticed that sometimes when I have pain and am lying down, she will balance on me, or drape herself over me. It's like a little heating pad.

BA: I just felt like she had tremendous healing ability. I remember that I kept saying, "You're quite the healer!" And she appeared to me to enjoy being seen for who she truly is.

CV: Well that's really cool. She likes being recognized and they definitely recognized you. They come and greet everybody but I think you're getting special greetings.

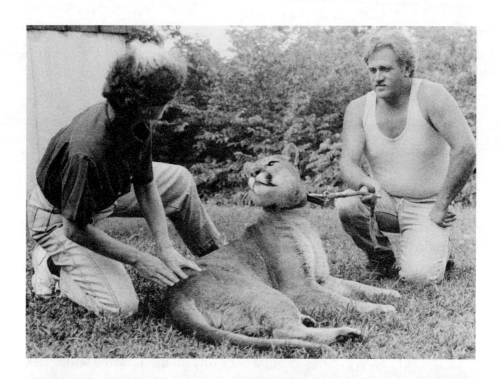

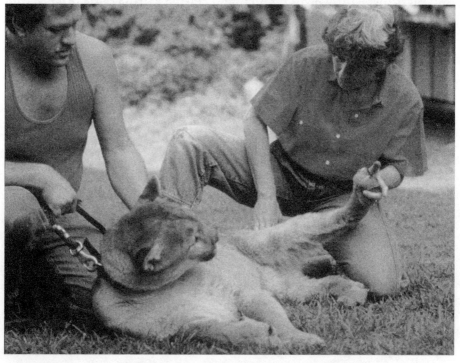

Top. *Brent on alert, but allowing me to proceed.* **Bottom.** *Brent cautious, but allowing me to work with him. Photos by Roy Inman.*

Deep Connection Transforms Aggression

Briah Anson writes about her work with Brent, a mountain lion

A few years ago I had the opportunity to do some Rolfing® Structural Integration on a mountain lion. This full grown two-year-old male weighed approximately 185 pounds. I was curious as to how he would respond to this kind of touch. Would he be calm as I worked? What would be the short and long term effects?

Brent had been raised by his owner, Pete, since he was a small cub. When Brent was close to a year old he became quite destructive inside the house as well as a bit dangerous to Pete and his family. Occasionally he would come up and take Pete by surprise, slap his head and knock him across the room. Pete realized that it was time to build Brent a large room of his own outside. The cute, playful cub was now a growing mountain lion that could inadvertently cause quite a lot of damage.

The prospect of even being close to an animal of this type appealed to me so I ventured out with an attitude of, "Well, let's see what happens." Pete didn't know anything about Rolfing SI and seemed pretty skeptical about any changes that might occur.

A year previous to this, Pete had taken Brent out of his large cage to have some photographs taken with him. Brent would have nothing to do with this event. He kept lunging at the photographer and was determined to get him. Pete had put Brent back in his cage and had not worked with him at all since then.

Pete remarked, "Before Brent was Rolfed he would always want to grab you. He would hiss and growl and show his aggressive nature. If you walked up to his cage he would slap at you through the cage. You were definitely live prey. If a stranger came around, he would be bouncing off the walls. He was always wanting to get someone."

The First Session

Session one was conducted with great care and some quick jumps away from Brent. The Rolfing work started with his hindquarters as this seemed like the safest place to begin. However, Pete and his wife warned me that he absolutely hated having anyone mess with his hindquarters as he was very touchy and sensitive there. Nevertheless, I wasn't going to get any closer to that ferocious, growling mouth of his, so I opted to just take my time and do little bits of work as Brent permitted.

The session was touch-and-go for about the first hour-and-a-half. After that Brent was so relaxed and in such an altered state that I was able to work around his head and jaws. There were even a few moments when I was able to lie on Brent and he seemed to be just fine with that. It wasn't until someone walked behind us that he quickly turned his head and was back on full alert. It was then that I realized that Brent was fully accepting the Rolfing work and me. A deeply connected bond had been established between us.

Two weeks later I returned and Pete reported that Brent was a different cat. He remarked that the day he had his session he was so mellow that Pete just kept going out to the cage and hanging out with him. "I wanted to take full advantage of this time with him as I figured it would wear off by the next day." The surprise continued as Brent remained very calm and mellow all week. "It's like you took the aggression out of him," Pete said. His appetite increased dramatically, by two-thirds his normal intake for a couple of weeks, and then leveled off.

The Second Session

I was curious as to whether Brent would recognize me when I returned for my second visit. I came with three friends who approached the cage, and Brent just remained in a crouched, watchful posture. A few minutes later I approached the cage. He instantly jumped up at the cage and greeted me with a half-hearted growl/hiss. He then threw himself down on the ground and rolled over on his back. He definitely remembered me and the reaction was positive.

Session two proceeded as if Brent was good and ready. He just crouched down and started chewing on the lead rope that Pete had around his neck like a dog busy chewing on a bone. Within thirty minutes, Brent was definitely in an altered state and extremely relaxed.

Within an hour's time, I was literally holding his head and opened his lip just to see if I could work his gums. Much to my surprise he responded as if I had administered an anesthetic. I was holding his head and he simply dropped the full weight of it into my hands. And so concluded the second session.

The Third Visit

I did not return to see Brent again for another six weeks. I couldn't believe my eyes. Brent, already fully grown, was longer in length by about two inches and larger overall in body size. Pete had managed to give him a bath earlier in the day. This task took some assistance and quite some time. Pete said it left Brent on the mad side. Pete was a little apprehensive as to how Brent might respond to a Rolfing session this time. He was a little frisky and there were certainly some moments of caution, but once again there was a welcoming acceptance of me and of the Rolfing work.

There was a professional photographer along on this trip, and he made some very interesting observations. He reported that he was fascinated watching Brent's eyes as I worked. He described it this way, "Amphibians have a transparent second eyelid and one stays open and the other closes while they swim underwater. It seemed as though Brent had a similar phenomenon occurring; the outer eye would remain open and stationary and then there would be an internal blink behind the eye—like a shutter that would open and close for about a tenth of a second. His eyes looked very filmy and would become more moist as Briah continued working on him. The blinks ceased as he got more relaxed and the pupils continued to dilate. He would just get a blank stare. This would remain for a period of time and every once in a while he would come out of this trance state, look around, and be focused once again."

Observations

The happy part of this whole lion adventure is that Pete is once again able to have contact with Brent and is now planning on building a larger cage where he can start training and working with Brent.

After his second Rolfing session, Pete took Brent to his nephew's school and the seventh grade class was able to be close to Brent. Of course, Pete had Brent in a small traveling cage and the children were able to pet him on his back through the bars. Brent seemed to be at ease with this encounter, and needless to say, the children were thrilled.

It seems as though the possibilities for Brent's future and Pete's interaction with him have been facilitated in such a way as to provide more joy for both of them.

In terms of the Rolfing process, I worked with him in much the same way as I would a human body, facilitating balance and finding the line.

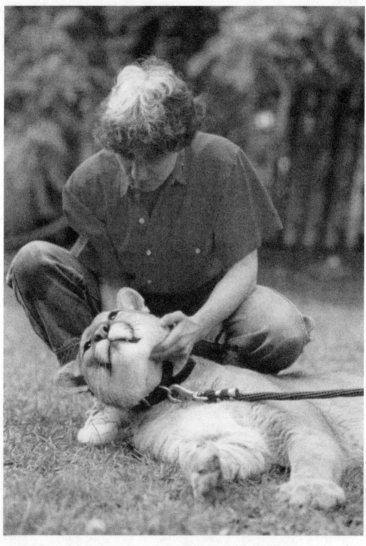

Brent in a trance state during his third and last session, totally opening to the power of Rolfing® SI. Photo by Roy Inman.

The difference is that, being a four-legged creature, Brent has two vertical lines. The fascial tissue responded similarly to human fascia. After the Rolfing sessions he appeared longer, more balanced, and was walking and moving more easily and rhythmically. Since working with Brent, I have been very fortunate to have many experiences like this with the animals that live with us and are willing to teach us about themselves.

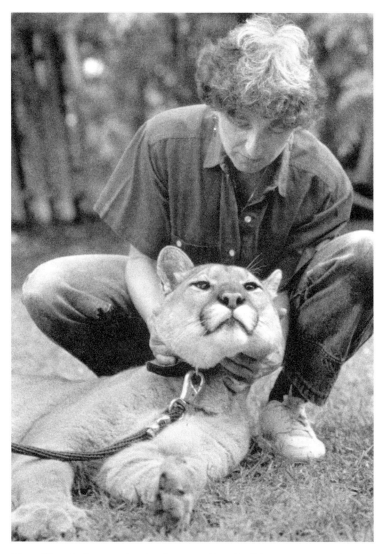

The ultimate human/animal connection. In this rare moment, through Rolfing® SI, I experienced an amazing sense of oneness and mutual trust. Photo by Roy Inman.

Even Roosters?

Rowan Scherf, on her rooster, Liam

Liam, a young rooster, lived with our family, which included several humans, several dogs, and Liam's two brothers, Jense and Malcolm. The roosters were beginning to mature when I was getting the Rolfing® series from Briah. We talked a lot about what kind of animals she had Rolfed, and I remember asking her if she had ever worked on snakes, birds, or carnivores. Following an impulse, I had to ask: "Have you ever Rolfed a chicken?"

I was astonished to find out that she hadn't. I mean, Briah had Rolfed a moose, giant cats, and everything in between . . . why not a chicken?

Out of a mixture of curiosity and an impulse to experiment, we decided to have Briah do a Rolfing session one of my roosters. Since I had a better bond with Liam than I had with the other two, I decided to choose him. My dad and I brought Liam in to St. Paul to see Briah.

The next part of the story is hard to explain. With Rolfing, the Rolfer™ has to get their hands deep into the muscles, and most people would freak out at the thought of getting their hands into a rooster with sharp claws. Fortunately, Briah has a gift with animals, and Liam remained quite calm. He seemed to understand that her intention was to help him, like this was a good thing in the long run. He behaved as perfectly as a rooster could, and more, during the session.

The results were easy to see. Before the session, the three roosters were almost identical. Now, Liam has a coat shinier than the others, and his gentle manner makes the other roosters seem like brigands. Whenever I go into the chickens' pen I sit in the middle, and Liam hops onto my lap, nudging my hand to make me pet him. We have nicknamed the other roosters Shark and Fighter, because whenever we come into the pen, they try to attack us.

Liam, however, always remains the lady's gentleman: calm, sweet-tempered, good-natured, self-assured; unusual traits to find in a rooster. He moves with a grace and demeanor that has elevated him to the stature of alpha rooster in his threesome. But he remains kind to the hens, for which they are most grateful. And Briah has now filled that chicken-gap in her repertoire of animals she's done Rolfing work on.

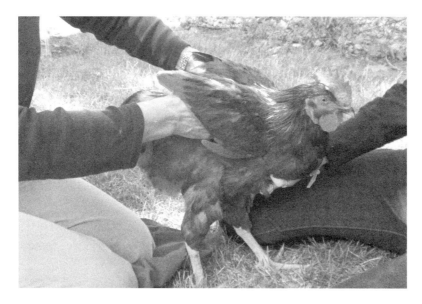

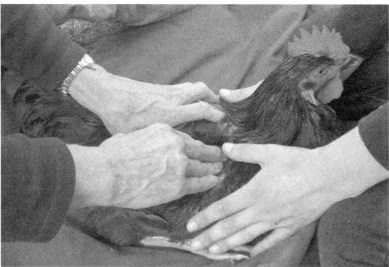

Top. *While I had both hands under his wings and well into his body, Liam, cooperated by stretching his head and neck out from his shoulders.*
Bottom. *Liam calm and relaxed during the session.*

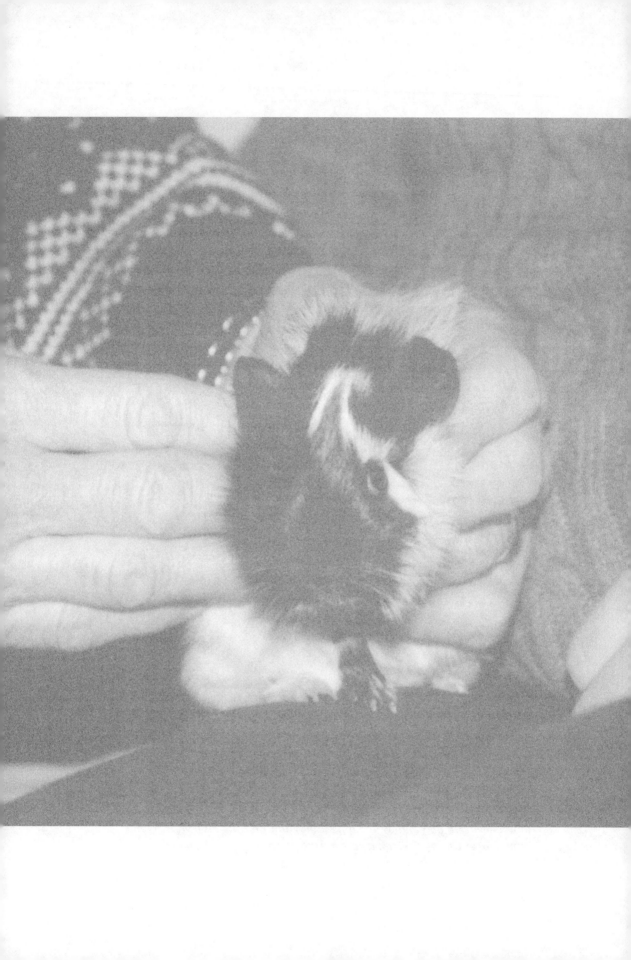

Issues Arising from Pet Rescue and Trauma

▶ *Physical health and mental health: it's the same thing.*

▶ *The body process is not linear, it's circular; always, it is circular. One thing goes awry and its effects go on and on. A body is a web, connecting everything with everything.*

▶ *If you want a different conclusion, start with a different premise.*

DR. IDA P. ROLF, from *Ida Rolf Talks about Rolfing and Physical Reality*, Rosemary Feitis, ed., Harper Row: NY; 1978

An Introductory Conversation Between Deborah Thayer, Movement Educator, and Briah Anson, Certified Advanced Rolfer™

Deborah Thayer: I am a dancer, choreographer, dance/somatic movement educator, and movement therapist. I've been in the Movement field for thirty years. I've had Rolfing® Structural Integration several times, including sessions with Rosemary Feitis, Tyr Thorn, and Briah Anson. I met Briah eight years ago. She has worked on many of my pets. The thing that I think is most significant about Briah's work is that it doesn't hurt! Briah's approach to the body is to be in alignment with the systems of the body. This enables her to tune in to what the whole system needs, enter into each system as it needs, and integrate the whole body.

She has an intelligence about how she works. I don't know whether this is an energetic intelligence or an intelligence of her hands and her touch but she is able to access particular systems so accurately that she doesn't need to press hard and muscle her way through the body. Her touch has a lot of finesse and accuracy to it. This helps the body easily assimilate information from her touch. It's like using a laser light instead of a big flashlight. This specificity of touch and intention enables her to work into you as an entire person—not a body that needs ABC or has symptoms ABC. She's trained to see the whole picture and this might be why she is able to use homeopathy accurately as well.

I think Briah is naturally attracted to putting her hands on animals. I remember saying to her once, "How can you do that? You don't really know the anatomy, do you?" And she said, "You don't really need to." Instead, she has this gift of being able to sense the entire character, personality, and life force coming through each type of body. She's then able to treat the whole body. Knowing the anatomy is wholly secondary to this type of intelligence. What do you think, Briah?

Briah Anson: I think that there is an anatomy of form that I am able to see. I am able to see gait problems. I'm able to feel where they are tied up, what needs to be released and how it needs to be released. Then I work in layers to accomplish that so they can have better function. I see it; I feel it in my hands; I can also see it when they move, in the same way that you can, Deborah, as a movement specialist.

I know that a four-legged will have two sets of vertical lines that I'm organizing through the body, aligning the energy from the ground up through the legs right up into the shoulder, or right up into the pelvis. Then drawing a midline up through the torso, neck and head—it really becomes a sculpting process.

It is science and art coming together.

Cats as Teachers:
Integrating Structure, Movement, and Being

A conversation between Deborah Thayer and Briah Anson

Deborah Thayer: Let's start with Behemoth MonChiChi. All my cats have been from the streets. B had a really hard time. I think he got hit by a car. He was very underweight, his coat was short, matted down, and a dirty yellow. We'd seen him outside for about half a year and had been feeding him. We knew his original owners and they'd let him out on the street. One day he was sitting at my door looking up at me for about an hour. I said "That's it; I can't take it anymore!" and scooped him up into my arms and threw him in my bedroom. He started purring right away. He was so appreciative to come inside, I think. We took him to the vet. His whole back end had been scratched up. His right leg would swing out to the side in a very strange gait.

Briah Anson: B had been hit from the left side and the force of the impact on the soft tissue threw his right hip out. So he could not move through himself, he had to swing the right leg out and around in order to propel himself forward.

DT: Technically, there was lateral flexion in the pelvis, so the right side was condensed, the left leg was expanded and the right leg would swing posteriorly, then laterally, and he'd make a half circle with the leg.

BA: He had to walk "around himself," such was the force of the impact. Basically, he had a hitch in his git-a-long.

DT: Seeing this poor dear cat suffering, I thought to myself, Briah can work on him. And she did right away. All I had to do was say "Look at this poor cat, Briah!"

BA: I started with the front end, to create some space in the chest and through the shoulders, so that as he moved with his front legs, his rear legs could propel themselves through the front. I had to free up the shoulder girdle first. It was obvious to me too, that the hind end was so condensed and compacted that he must have been hit by a car.

DT: I think you did two full sessions and a few mini sessions. His hips did come out of that lateral flexion to be more in line with his shoulder girdle.

BA: You could draw a midline through the middle of his head and all the way back through his spine—he was starting to line up.

DT: He couldn't jump very well initially. Our window ledges are about four feet high. He'd attempt to jump onto them and end up sliding down the wall. It was awful to watch; he had no strength. Now he jumps up and down and all around. Not only that, but his fur just went "POOF." It's now a big, long, white, gorgeous, luxurious coat. So the combination of love, nutrition and the Rolfing gave him his life back.

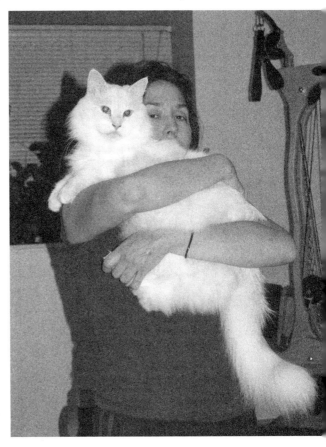

Behemoth Monchichi with Deborah, his mom, who says: "It was the combination of love, nutrition, and Rolfing® SI that gave him his life back."

BA: This is due to the increased circulation, oxygen, blood flow, and creating space in the layers of tissue. This creates a sense of space and lightness in the body.

DT: I hate to say it but he also became more of a badass. He was starting to feel his oats; he got really confident. Around the house he became more dominant with the other cats. After the work, he got much bigger. He's like a polar bear now; he has this polar bear essence. I think this is probably why it took three months for his name to come to me. He was changing, his character was changing as he was getting heavier and becoming more himself.

BA: I'd like to add that one of the goals of the Rolfing process is to evoke the potential or the true essence of the being. I think this fits in with Deborah's experience. In B's traumatized state he could not express the being that he was, hence, it was difficult for Deborah to find the appropriate name.

DT: His original name was Ghost. How appropriate was that! At the time he was ghost-like. None of the names we called him stuck.

BA: Until the structural work was resolved. At that point, it seemed, you naturally and intuitively came to name him. The name Behemoth MonChiChi is a big name! This cat is not fat, but he has a largeness and a large personality. Deborah, what did you discover about B's name?

DT: My sister googled it and learned that MonChiChi is a Japanese cartoon character that's really mischievous and furry. It stands on two legs, but, it is very cat-like. I was amazed that it matched him so perfectly.

BA: I think Deborah has described the Rolfing effects very well. I had the intention, during those two major sessions to free him up and to align him structurally. Then, with the passing of weeks he was able to find his own line and to integrate and start getting that rear leg under himself and moving better. The additional five or ten minutes here or there helped him advance even more, to the point that when all the sessions were complete his gait was almost normal. This was a small cat that was hit by a large car so it was quite a major traumatic event. To see him move now and lunge from the floor straight up onto the counter from standing still shows a tremendous change in his ability to contract and expand his muscles. He knows exactly how and where to land to not knock over the plants. And he does it very gracefully.

DT: It's true—like any strong, healthy cat would be able to do. He also did this really wild thing once. He was on the windowsill which is about four feet from the floor. One of my clients was on my Gyrotonic machine. He flew from the windowsill about five feet on the diagonal onto the floor in front of my client. We couldn't believe it! He just FLEW. You can imagine a little cat or a sprightly cat doing this, but, this was a big huge cat, flying through the air in front of our faces. We were both impressed! He landed "KERTHUNK." He's a big cat and he can absorb that impact.

BA: I think that speaks to the work also, as he is able to absorb that impact in his tissues and does not then walk away limping.

DT: He does it all the time. He leaps off of things. He doesn't just crawl down things; he soars!

BA: An animal that's not healthy is not going to be experimental in that way, is not going to be taking those kinds of chances.

DT: He can move weights and open doors. He'll put his paw under the door and yank. He's a real strong cat. He must have been genetically very strong.

BA: He must have been, but he had been compromised. What the work did was release the trauma so that his nature could unfold.

DT: Which is interesting, because Paris, our other cat, went in an entirely opposite direction. He, too, was hit by a car. Paris was an overly aggressive, totally feral cat. It took us about two years to train him to be socialized. He was an aggressive bully. We did a lot of work with Dr. Pomeroy, our veterinarian, in St. Paul.

BA: He does CRA, Contact Reflex Analysis. It is a system of applied kinesiology that gets at what is going on nutritionally, mentally and emotionally. It's used with humans as well.

DT: We had Paris working with Dr. Pomeroy at the same time that Briah was Rolfing him. Paris looked to me like he was pretty much intact. But, once you started Rofling him, he suddenly got really uptight and started hissing.

BA: Almost like a defensive/aggressive gesture.

DT: His whole body tightened up. Briah kept at it and I remember the moment when she seemed to be hit by some information and she knew he'd been hit by a car. Briah kept going in there and I would stabilize him as she worked.

BA: Deborah would hold his head because I didn't want to get my hands bitten or scratched. Paris was experiencing quite a bit of pain and trauma. Some of it felt like trauma in the present tense and some of it felt like it was releasing old trauma. There was also a lot of fear associated with the work I was doing.

DT: The most significant change was not so much structural but behavioral—his personality changed. All he wants to do now is be held and loved. We don't see that bully any more. He'd also scream a lot. At one point, we had to put him in a three foot by four foot cage to isolate him from the other cats because he was terrorizing them.

BA: It was so obviously a painful place to be for Paris. He expressed it by bullying the other cats in the house in a very aggressive way. Frankly, I remember being a little afraid to work with him. He was fast and I was afraid of getting bitten or scratched. I was relying on Deborah to hold him down and hold his head to stabilize him. She wasn't using force, but I wanted to make sure that I wasn't feeling fearful as I worked on him because I needed to feel relaxed. That would enable me to free the layers very gently, gradually, confidently and carefully, and not be tense myself which would be communicated through my touch. I did three sessions with Paris, spaced about a month apart. It seemed to both of us that he was getting more comfortable in himself and more comfortable with what we were doing. He wasn't trying to hide from us.

DT: He was getting braver. He was always skittish around people. It took us two years to get him socialized after we took him off the streets. He lived in the study and wouldn't come out from underneath the desk while we were in the room for about three months. We couldn't touch him for several months. If we advanced toward him with our fingertips he would freak out. I had to come toward him with my face which he seemed to trust. It was kind of scary, coming literally face to face with a wild animal, but that's how we gained his trust, by me and my sister being that vulnerable. He'd probably been hit. He hates men.

BA: Well, those are clues that there was some abuse.

DT: And now he's our Paris Love-Bug. He's still skittish around people that he doesn't know but he's not skittish around me. And he LOVES my sister. As far as Paris is concerned, she is his mate, or his person. He wants love above food.

BA: I go over to Deborah's every week for a movement lesson. Paris is around; he doesn't hide from me; he's not skittish; he seems very much in his body. He seems confident; doing what he wants to do.

DT: He still doesn't like men though. When I have male clients he'll go into another room. So here is Behemoth MonChiChi becoming more expansively dominant and Paris becoming more loving and gentle. Two contrasting personality shifts.

BA: Truly, each of them becoming more of who they are. I think this is a major point of how the work intervenes in that way. The work did not impose a template on them. The Rolfing process helped bring their personalities out, their spirits, their essential natures.

DT: I think what's really interesting about Structural Integration is that it's never working with a separate entity. When you work on the structure, you work on the movement. And when the body moves it also frees up the emotion, intelligence, and essence of the being. I think it is impossible to work on the structure and not affect those things.

I see a couple of these same things in dance. As some structures free up I see the dancers integrating new information in their bodies. Often there's a lot of emotional release and they become more of themselves. I also see women who are in their forties or fifties who haven't done a lot of movement and have a lot of stored emotion. When they start to move all of this surfaces and there can be huge emotional releases. We try to calm their systems down a little so they can function in the world again. It's really great to work with Briah, because sometimes with movement you can't get at it; someone needs to go into the structure manually and free it up.

BA: And other times you need movement patterns to re-educate the structure as to the potential that has been freed up. Because of how peoples' brains are wired they don't realize that they are so much more capable of moving with more options.

DT: That's right. Once you free up the structure you don't want that person to keep moving in their old habitual ways. That would take the structure back to where it was previously. You want to help it find a different way to move.

BA: We have to rewire the habitual patterns. Now that the structure is freed up and capable of moving differently, we have to retrain the brain to know that it has a different way of doing things that is much more efficient and easy. This is how we work together. We have collaborated for eight years with countless clients.

I have seen Deborah once a week for the last three years. Part of my story is I that I did ballet two to three times a week from the time I was eight years old until I was eighteen. That is a lot of formative years of hammering and holding patterns. On top of that I was a severe asthmatic from age eight until twenty-six, which accentuated the patterns that were there from ballet. So it's taken a lot of Rolfing® work and a lot of movement work with Deborah to have my body "get" that it can let go. The evolution of structure takes a lot of time and consciousness. With animals, who have an innate intelligence, they have a more instinctual response. Although they have mental and emotional problems from what has happened to them, they are able to take a little bit of work and reorganize themselves at a quantum speed compared to humans.

I haven't been around cats a lot but I have been most impressed with cats and their ability to regenerate from trauma. It's faster than most animals that I've worked on. It's a gift; it's part of how they are innately wired. The beautiful thing about watching these cats that have been through the Rolfing process is that it's inherent in them to be able to move gracefully and stay soft. When they need explosive movement and power they know how to do the contraction and expansion in a nanosecond. We can learn this from watching them. They don't live with intentional patterns.

DT: That's why it's good to have them around the studio. They stretch and yawn their movements through all their limbs and parts. You never see them isolating an arm. Everything is always being integrated into the entire system, the whole body.

BA: As a movement therapist, this is what Deborah is trying to help us humans learn and express. That when one part moves everything else is moving in concert with the other parts with grace and resilience.

DT: That's why, when people work out in a gym and they isolate the muscles and stabilize the spine, it's probably one of the worst things for bodies. Bodies are not wired to do that. There's nothing in life that replicates that movement. A lot of repetitive movements, like on the pecs for instance, pulls other muscles out of balance. People are then set up for injury when they do something innocuous like grab something off a shelf or close a door . . .

One set of fibers are overly developed and others have not been coordinating with them in an intelligent way. So the body gets pulled out of balance. We have to do activities that we are neurologically wired for. For instance, the brachiation pattern that we are wired to do—we build upon that by going rock climbing. This activity uses all the structures and dimensions in the body with that reach and pull, reach and pull. We have to use our eyes, touch, fingers, weight, the entire spine, the push through the legs. This is how a balanced body gets developed. Cats do that instinctively. They move with their whole body. You can see it all the way through the tail.

BA: As humans, we tend to isolate the parts of our structures.

DT: I think it's a function of modern day life. As a cave person, I think you would look with your entire body at the water buffalo that you want to eat for dinner. It's a whole body experience. This is a lesson we can learn from our companion animals. I use the cats as an example of how to move, "push through the feet as if you were kneading like a cat." People get that movement.

BA: In conclusion, cats are our teachers?

DT: Yes! And a cat that has had Rolfing is an even better teacher because they integrate the movement into their systems.

The Emotionally Challenged Shelter Dog

Beth Miller, on her dogs, Bronte and Birdie

Birdie is a seven-month-old puppy that I rescued from an animal shelter. They told me that she is a Pointer-Spaniel mix. She had been in two agencies by the time I rescued her, so she was very, very far behind in some social and developmental skills. She was fearful of everything. She had never even been exposed to grass. She didn't know how a door worked. She had never been on a leash. She didn't know what stairs were. So I started at ground zero with her and she has come along beautifully. She is not afraid of dogs anymore, even though she just got attacked by one. She is still very shy around strangers; it takes her a long time to warm up to a person, but once you've gained her trust, she is very affectionate, loyal, and friendly.

I had gone through the ten sessions of Rolfing® with Briah several years ago, and then sent my daughter for sessions. We have both done continuing work, and I even had my elderly dog, Bronte, a big Chesapeake who passed away a couple of years ago, get Rolfed.

Bronte's Story

Bronte had been a very active dog. Chesapeakes are built for stamina and I utilized that to the utmost. We ran, snow shoed, and hiked. She was tireless and developed hip dysplasia, and became incredibly arthritic. Vets told me I might get nine years with Bronte at the most and that they couldn't believe she was as functional as she was. But Bronte lived to be almost thirteen and I really believe that it was the Rolfing that helped make that happen.

Bronte was seven or eight years old at the time I first brought her in to see Briah. She had been having a lot of difficulty with her arthritis. She was slowing down, which older dogs do, but knowing what the Rolfing did for me, I thought that it might help her move easier in her later years—and I think it did!

We did a half dozen sessions at least, and we did them in a pretty timely fashion, once a month for about six months. She responded really well during the sessions, and it seemed to help her mobility quite a bit. I found it interesting that even though Bronte had been a very well adjusted dog, she really settled into her own in her senior years. That's when she became more connected to people, to me, and to clients. She was connected on another level than is usual for a dog, and my clients noticed this. It was incredible.

I'm a massage therapist and I tend to do very deep specific work, which can be incredibly uncomfortable for people. Bronte would sleep in her little bed in my office and became attuned to my clients. When I would get into areas with my clients that were uncomfortable for them I wouldn't always pick up on it from them right away. A split second before it became clear to me, Bronte would either whine or come to my client and try to comfort them. They would often comment, "Oh, how does she know that this is really uncomfortable for me?" She just knew and she was very comforting. For a big, rather dominant dog, she was very nurturing during those sessions.

Bronte had been a therapy dog since she was about five, and had always been in my office with me. But until she got Rolfed, I hadn't seen this empathetic and tuned in side of her. She saw that as her work. Toward the end when she couldn't get down stairs very well by herself and could not get up stairs at all, at the start of the day I would just say, "just stay up here." She wanted to be in on it. She lived for that toward the end, and I felt that our work and the Rolfing helped Bronte and I bond. We had always been close. We worked together and played together, but once she had been Rolfed, it was like she was on a different level. It was fascinating to me.

Birdie's Turn

When you adopt a pet from a shelter, you never know what you're going to be getting, and adopting Birdie was a different experience than I'd had before. I usually felt an immediate connection with an animal, but with Birdie I didn't. She was so shy when I saw her in the shelter that I'm not sure what triggered it for me. I didn't have that emotional reaction, "Oh, I can't leave this dog here in this shelter, I just have to rescue her!" I don't know what it was that drew me to her because she wasn't giving me anything. She didn't act like she wanted to go home with me, but there was something there, and it's great to see more of that come out now, that little spark in there behind her eyes. But I knew that I wouldn't be able to help her bring that out on my own—she needed some intervention.

I didn't get Birdie with the intention of her being a therapy dog or tuning into my clients. I got her for companionship, but it would be so lovely if that kind of therapeutic relationship could come about. I took Birdie to see Briah a week after I got her so the Rolfing started fairly quickly. We did another session two weeks later, and the third one after another month. I'm looking forward to more sessions with her.

Birdie had been out of the shelter for only a week when she had her first session, and she was very shy and skittish with Briah. As the session went on, I saw her relax into the work. It seemed that even though

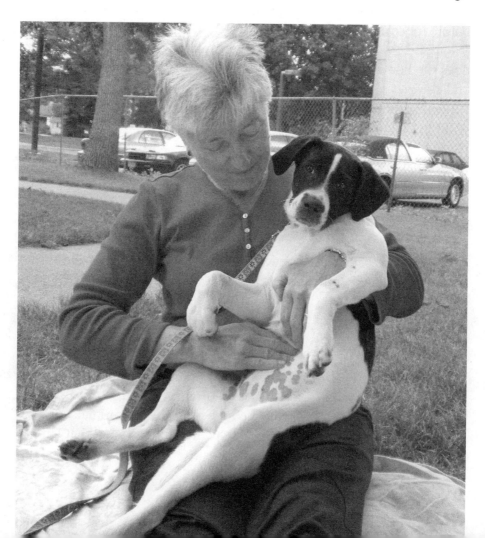

she looked very sound, she was a little bit disconnected with what dogs should do. She didn't know how to run and I had to teach her. She wasn't comfortable in her own skin. She wasn't connected at all to herself. I saw that start to change after the first session, and then with each subsequent session. I think it really helped her settle into herself, get comfortable with what a dog should do, and gain a little more confidence. She's still shy but at least she's willing to try things. I'm sure it's a combination of everything we've been doing—I work with her every minute I get and the positive reinforcement is helping as well. But I think there's only so much you can do. I think things have to happen at a cellular level and the Rolfing has expedited this process for her. I've even had people comment, "Boy, she's really coming out of this!" She really is. She's walking with a little swagger now and starting to settle into who she is. I'm hoping that continuing sessions will integrate her a little more and help her get over the crisis of confidence that she's suffered from.

The first time Briah watched her walk, we noticed that her left hind leg lagged behind. Her walk was very awkward as if she had been in a cage her whole life. She had no muscle tone—she was just a little waif. But even at the end of that first session, we could see her body starting to integrate itself. Her walk was beginning to track a little better. Her head was not swinging all over the place. She was starting to find her ground right after that first session.

With the other two sessions, her muscle development continued. I exercise her pretty rigorously and she's starting to develop some tone. I'm noticing more symmetry in her body. After the second session it was interesting to see a kind of a calm settle into her. After the third session she popped out of the shyness a little bit more. Perhaps her nervousness diminished after the first couple sessions, and then the shyness after the third. She was a little more confident after the third session.

I love to be outside exercising which is why I want an active dog. For the first six weeks, I literally had to drag Birdie down the street to go for a walk because she was terrified of everything. We built up to these walks very gently for the first few weeks. I slowly lengthened our walks, first to build up her body tone and tissue, and second to help her become desensitized to lawnmowers, little kids and strollers.

In one of my own Rolfing sessions with Briah I mentioned this fear, and Briah immediately said, "You know what, we need to give her a big boost to pass the fear." She recommended a particular homeopathic rem-

Opposite. *Birdie, a seven-month-old pointer-spaniel finally relaxing into the work.*

edy. I was at my wit's end because after six weeks, the neighbors were all laughing, "Oh, there's Beth dragging her dog down the street again, is this dog ever going to learn?" I said, "What kind of a dog doesn't want to go for a walk, my goodness! What am I gonna do with a dog that doesn't like to walk?" Briah had me get a strong dose of the homeopathic remedy. I gave it to her that evening, and the next morning she was prancing down the street. I mean literally *prancing* down the street. I kept waiting for her old fears to kick in: "Uh-oh, I'm supposed to be shy and hold back and pull back," but she has never done it since.

Of course I overdid that first walk, but she was no worse for the wear. She's excited to go for walks now. It's not just that she's going along for it, she's leading the charge out the door, and she's loving it! It would have been interesting to see what would have happened without the Rolfing and the homeopathy—to see if she would have progressed like she has. All I know is that in the last three months she has progressed amazingly well.

Briah says that in Rolfing animals it is so much easier to break through the mental and emotional barriers than with people. Three sessions can be a lot of input for an animal, and she's growing with that. We knew Birdie had a lot of emotional baggage from being in the shelter and from whatever got her there. She had a rough beginning and I'm thrilled to see her come as far as she has. I don't think we'd be where we are today without the Rolfing. These shelter dogs often have a lot of trauma and most people don't know how to handle them. People get frustrated and without knowing what to do it can often result in more abuse for the animal. You can't treat a really shy dog in the same way as a dog like Bronte who was just full bore ahead. I probably could have whacked Bronte over the head to get her attention and she wouldn't have blinked. But with Birdie I use very gentle corrections because she's more fragile and I don't know how she will take it. Not knowing her background, the stock she came from, her history, or predispositions, I feel it's very important for her to get the Rolfing. It's helping her become as sound as she can, both mentally and physically.

Homeopathy Treatments

Briah gave me the name of a vet who is also a classical homeopath that we thought might help Birdie with her emotional and mental weaknesses. Birdie had just been attacked by another dog, so the vet had to treat her for that first. Our first visit was a traditional vet visit because of the dog bite, but I want to eventually treat Birdie fairly aggressively with homeopathy. The vet did give me a remedy to help Birdie with her nervousness on the second visit.

When Briah had recommended the homeopathic remedy I was kind of leary but thought, "oh, okay, it's worth a try." I was blown away by the quick turnaround and how much immediate impact that had for Birdie. That encouraged me to continue with homeopathic treatments.

The vet wants to work on the level of her physiology right now. Birdie developed a tumor on her leg which we are still exploring and the vet is using probiotics and fish oils to boost her immune system and give her what may have been lacking in her shelter diet. Puppy chow in the shelter isn't exactly nutritious. The vet has given Birdie another homeopathic constitutional remedy. Perhaps once her physiology gets stronger, more of her picture homeopathically will emerge in terms of what she needs next. So it is kind of an unwinding, it's a progression.

I'm continuing to work with Birdie by constantly training and exposing her to more of the outside world. We are starting obedience training tomorrow! I see her growth as a lifelong thing with the Rolfing and homeopathy as a big part of that. I hadn't learned about Rolfing when Bronte was young so she did not have the benefit of that until she was pretty old. I have really high hopes that Birdie will be able to live a long full life because I got her started so early with both these treatments. We all know that you have to have a healthy physical side to support the emotional side, so it all goes hand in hand.

Looking Back

As far as Birdie participating in my massage practice the way Bronte used to do, well, she was terrified of the clients at first. She would run away and hide, then she graduated to standing and barking, and then she managed to bark and wag her tail. In the last few weeks, she just runs downstairs and sits by their chair and waits for their treat. People like to give her treats, but she doesn't let them pet her yet. At first I kept her in her kennel while I was working on clients, and now she just crawls into her bed and goes to sleep while I work. She just knows that that's what we do, and that's her job. She hasn't interacted yet with clients. Occasionally at the end of the day when she's getting bored, she'll try to put her paws up on the table or sniff their hair, but when I tell her to lay down, she goes right back. She walks them up to the door and wags her tail good-bye, so I've seen a huge improvement in that. I think part of the problem is that I live alone so she only sees other people for a few minutes—she'll walk them in, then sleep for the session and walk the clients out again. I don't think she has enough exposure to make the connections that might bring her out of her shyness. She needs a pack, if you will, rather than just me.

She is coming along beautifully, and has become very connected to my daughter and my parents. It took her a long time. They don't live here so I've been making trips to see them so that Birdie can stay connected. I had a client that came very regularly and has since moved, but Birdie really connected with this client. She seems to connect with cat people more than dog people, because cat people know that you don't get in a cat's face—they will walk away. So they tend to sit back a little further and let her come to them. Birdie responds much better to that than people moving toward her with a high-pitched voice and wanting to reach out and pet. There's a client who is a cat person. She said that she didn't even know how to act around dogs. I hadn't seen her for a month when she came back to town for a session with me. Birdie remembered her and was very affectionate. She seems to be remembering and that's an improvement.

My daughter took care of Birdie at her house shortly after I got her for four days. Then just ten days later, Haley came over and Birdie was too shy to go to her. Haley's comment was, "Hey honey, you pooped on my floor! Come on, we bonded, where are you?" It took about ten minutes for Birdie to warm up to her, but now, after Birdie's treatments she gets excited to see Haley and picks right back up where she left off. So I'm seeing some memory retention now and being able to sustain the trust that she develops with a person.

Briah says that sustaining trust is a very important sign of resolving trauma in humans, and it takes awhile. In only three months, the progress Birdie has made is unbelievable. I hadn't expected her to be this far along with her physical and emotional development after only three months out of the shelter. She deserves some of the credit too, because she's trying to embrace things in her own way. She's starting to trust a little more.

I think the Rolfing kept Bronte alive a couple more years than she would have had without it and it was a good quality of life. It's been very interesting to lead a dog through the final stages of her life with that

Rolfing experience, and to now get the opportunity to give a young dog this experience and watch her progress through her whole life. It's really rewarding to watch that progression over time. I got to see Bronte go out with it, and Birdie start her life with it.

I sent several of my clients to Briah after I'd taken them as far as I could. What I found interesting is that the selling point for them was not that I had been Rolfed, or that my daughter had been, but that Bronte had gone through it. They all said something like, "Well, if it was good enough for Bronte, it's good enough for me!" The fact that Rolfing crossed lines beyond the human experience, that this was a universal way to treat not just animals but people, got through to them.

I think there was an element of fear about Rolfing because they'd heard it would be really painful and uncomfortable, and that you might go through some real life changing experiences. It can be all of that, but maybe it was less intimidating knowing that Bronte went through it, and it wasn't painful and she not only survived but thrived. Many of my clients have been with me since the beginning of my practice which is twelve years, and they could see how much better Bronte's quality of life was. Bronte was a kind of living testimonial. I could talk about it, but they could see it in Bronte. They could see that she lived a lot longer than was predicted and that she lived well.

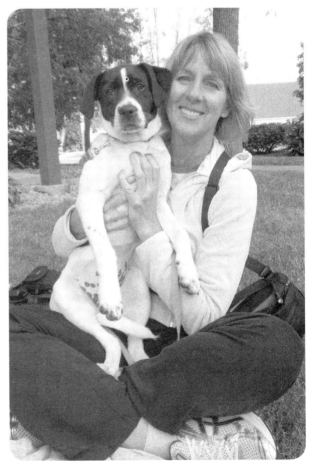

Birdie, now emotionally bonded with her owner Beth.

Rescuing the Rescue Cat

Jessica Phillps, on her Devon rex, Oscar

I had been doing the Rolfing® series for the past several months for myself because of severe muscle tension, TMJ (temporomandibular joint dysfunction), neck and back problems, and lots of digestive problems from Crohn's disease and food allergies. I had a lot of improvement and toward the end of those sessions I began to wonder if it would help my cat Oscar, who is twelve years old and throws up about five times a week on my bed. That's been going on for four out of the five years I've had Oscar.

I've taken him to the vet a number of times, and they said that it's normal for cats to throw up. My vet said, in fact, he had a cat that threw up every week and that that was okay. But because I don't feel well when I throw up, I figured Oscar can't feel well when he does either. Sometimes it was undigested food but sometimes it was more digested food but a lot of bile with it. I tried a number of things that didn't work. Sometimes there were hairballs coming up too, so I brushed him every day and gave him hairball treats. I bathed him once a week and I started giving him some natural wet cat food hoping it would help with the digestion, but that didn't seem to do anything either. I've taken him to the vet three times just for that problem.

Introducing Oscar

Oscar is a Devon rex. They're very curious. They're playful. They're known for their kittenlike antics. They like to help you, be with you, help you do what you're doing. They are very inquisitive and they're a very, very active breed. They like to be up high, and he jumps onto counters, cupboards and into windows. Even though he is twelve years old, he's still very active. Devon rexes usually live to be about twenty-three. I have another cat, Cinnabar, who is five years younger. They run around and play, but Oscar can still do everything that Cinnabar can do. They're a very active breed, they talk a lot, and they're obsessed with food.

Oscar was always crying for food, always, day and night. Even if he'd just eaten he still cried for food—begging at his dish and walking around. He'd come up to me and paw and paw and paw until I gave him food. Even when I just tried to give him attention, thinking that's what he wanted, he'd run away to his dish. He doesn't want the attention, he just wants the food. That's been going on the whole time I've had him.

Oscar is a rescue cat. He was rescued from a home that had too many animals and then he was sent to the pound, then the Humane Society took him, and then Second Chance Animal Rescue took him, and they put him into a foster home until a permanent home could be found. I remember reading his profile and he just sounded like a wonderful cat, and I had to meet him. When I did go to meet him, the woman that was fostering him said that he was aggressive toward the other cats. He sat on top of his cat post and would jump on and attack any cat that walked by. During the day when she was at work, she had to lock up all the other cats in a bedroom so that Oscar didn't terrorize them. But I took one look at him and I said, "Let's go home, Oscar!"

Oscar starts Rolfing SI sessions

It was about a month ago that I brought him in for his first Rolfing session. Usually when I take him anywhere he doesn't like the kennel I bring him in. To get him out I have to take apart the entire kennel. I take off the top and the door, and then just lift him out of it because he won't walk out. But this time I opened the door and he ran right out onto the sheet in Briah's office. It shocked me, he'd never done that before unless he's at home. That was very uncharacteristic of him. He just took off out of there like he was ready, and he crouched down and we started to work. He wiggled a lot and he repositioned quite often, but he was enjoying it. I could tell his muscles were very tight and he had a hard time relaxing into the movement of it. But he didn't meow, didn't hiss, didn't show any aggressive behavior. There was no nipping, no hitting, but he was wagging his tail a lot, which is usually an indication of nervousness, so it was hard for him to relax.

Briah worked with him for at least an hour. As the hour progressed, he started to stretch out a little more. He started to focus his attention elsewhere in the room. Before that he was always looking to wherever Briah's hands were. He wasn't quite sure what was going on. He started to relax, lying down, moving and stretching his legs, lengthening himself. Toward the end of the session he started to move around a lot less, and he was almost falling asleep with his head in my hand.

One thing that surprised me during that first session was that he was very quiet, and he's usually a talker. He didn't say one peep, he was just taking it all in. I think it was very calming for him; he was really focusing and concentrating which helped him a lot. He's always been a very anxious cat. They're not an anxious breed, but because of his previous history where he may have been neglected, I think he developed this nervousness and aggression. But during this session he wasn't on edge or constantly crying.

At home that night and the next day, he was very quiet. In fact, a couple of times I went to look for him, wondering where he was, because normally I hear him somewhere. But no, he was just sitting quietly on the floor, looking around. He wasn't begging for food, he wasn't crying by his food dish, and when I went to pet him, he just sat there and enjoyed my hand on his back. He slept a lot that day, that night, and then the next day. I noticed his sleeping position looked different—he was more sprawled out. He's usually tightly curled in a little ball, but now he was spread out with a few paws up in the air. He was breathing more deeply, and he was really sleeping well. I think he was just processing the Rolfing session and letting everything settle in. The next day when I went to pick him up to give him a hug and a kiss, he just sat there and relaxed in my arms. Usually he'd jump right down and dart to his dish. I could already see lots of changes.

Usually Oscar and Cinnabar rough play quite a bit, and they weren't doing that as much. Oscar was just not taking part in it. He was very quiet, very relaxed, and they weren't biting, scratching and kicking each other. They usually tumble around, so that was different. It was quiet for quite a few days.

In the two weeks between Oscar's two Rolfing sessions, he hadn't thrown up on my bed. I had actually gone to get a waterproof mattress cover to put on my bed during the day because he was throwing up so much that I was having to wash all of my linens every day. I still put the cover on, but he didn't throw up, so that saved me quite a bit of time and stress over those two weeks. One of the cats had thrown up twice and I don't know which one it was, but it was just a small amount on the floor, so even if it was Oscar, it was a lot smaller than what it had been.

His feedings were going well. He didn't sit at his dish crying and begging for food, but he certainly reminded me when it was time! In between the feedings, he wasn't obsessed with his food dish. He used to obsessively lick his dish even when there was no food in it, and he hasn't been doing that.

The first couple of days, he didn't interact very much with Cinnabar, and I think he was catching up on sleep and readjusting. After that, they would play but it wasn't as rough. They have been sleeping together and snuggling a lot more, so those have been some positive changes. They're very different personalities. Cinnabar is hyper and he'll walk all over me when I'm sleeping. Oscar doesn't like that, and neither do I! Before the Rolfing, Oscar would chase Cinnabar off the bed, maybe biting or slapping him a couple times. Now Oscar just finds a different spot and goes back to sleep.

Two weeks later Briah did a second session, and I saw a lot of changes. Again, he walked right out of his cage when I opened the door in Briah's office. He walked onto the blanket and crouched down and we got to work. Briah didn't have to let him smell her hand or get used to her, she just dove right in, and he laid down and accepted everything. He didn't move as much. She worked deeper into the muscles, especially his back legs which were very tense. He's always been very protective of his rear and his hind legs and didn't like them touched. He didn't like his tail being touched either, so I was very surprised that he was so relaxed and let her work deeply into the muscle. He stretched his front paws and his back leg, and he didn't turn over to try to get to her, or flip over so she couldn't work on him.

She worked his abdominal area very deeply as well as the psoas, adductors, and his rotators. He remained there upside down with his front paws curled in the air and stayed in that posture. I could tell that he really enjoyed it. He had this look on his face like this session was way overdue. During the first session, he looked at me a lot making sure I was still there, but he didn't do that during this session. He was in a very meditative state. He stayed in one position for quite some time with his eyes getting smaller and starting to close.

Results

It's been another week since that last session, and I've noticed that one of the cats has thrown up on the floor once, but only a very small amount. He hasn't thrown up on my bed. He is eating a lot slower and not wolfing his food down. Often he'll eat a few pebbles, and then get a drink of water and wander back to his dish. He never took a water break while he was eating before. He is chewing all of his food, swallowing it, taking his time, breathing. So that's been quite a big difference.

When I pick him up, his back end used to just curl right up, and now when I pick him up, he's really relaxed and soft, and he just hangs in the air real flat and long and lean. His muscles are not nearly as tight as they were before. When I pet his back legs, or his back or tail, he doesn't

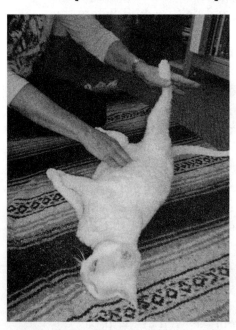

Oscar, taking to his Rolfing® SI session right away!

turn around and nip me. It's just like petting any other part of his body—he enjoys it. The muscle tightness must be so much less than it used to be, because there is no pain for him when I touch him or scratch his back. When I brush out his tail and his legs, he just stretches out for me now, instead of turning around to nip at me and run away.

He's moving differently too. He's been a lot quieter when he's running, and it's a lot more smooth. I used to hear a big thud when he jumped down, but now I don't. He's more graceful and balanced when he's jumping. His high leaps are much quicker now, too. I don't have any place in my apartment that he hasn't been able to get to: the top of the fridge, the microwave, my eight-foot wardrobe. Before the Rolfing he would have to sit and prepare himself for a high jump. He'd wait a moment, then wiggle his tail and then he'd jump. Now I just see this sudden flash of white. It's a jump up, down, and that's it, very fast.

He has stopped waking me up for food in the morning. When he heard the mail carrier, he would try to wake me up. It wasn't time for him to eat yet but that didn't matter to him. He would paw and paw, or he'd slap my forehead hard, and I'd put a pillow over my head. Then he would just stand on my back and tug my hair. He wouldn't give up. Then he would just cry, and cry, then jump on the floor where he'd rise up on his back feet, front paws in the air, screaming for food. But he hasn't done that in a very long time. He's sleeping through the night better.

It's obvious to me that his whole digestive system is working better. That's one of the benefits of Rolfing—that as we work to restructure the animal or the person, all the organs, all the muscles, and all the soft tissues start working better. I assume that he's assimilating and absorbing nutrition better and that's why he's not crying constantly for food. The Rolfing work has been the only change for him. I haven't changed his food, feeding times or anything else. It's helped tremendously—certainly turned his life around.

One of his ears used to get a lot of black waxy buildup and I had to give him prescription antibiotic ear drops. His right eye also oozes something reddish and I have to clean his eyes everyday and put in antibiotic drops. The vet said that was normal for their breed. Since the Rolfing, he hasn't had as much black waxy buildup and maybe that's also one of the Rolfing benefits, along with improved digestion, in that he is not having so many skin problems. He has always had blackheads on his tail. He has a stud tail is what they call it, and blackheads build up on those kinds of tails. I have to wash it off with peroxide shampoo. I'm hoping to keep seeing improvements in his skin and with the drainage in his eye so I can get him off of the antibiotic drops.

Briah thinks that at this point he is a good candidate for homeopathy, and I'm very interested in doing that for him. I've benefited from homeopathy, and there are no side effects, so I think that would be a great next step.

Adopting a Rescue Cat

The problem with rescue cats is that you never know their full history. I adopted Oscar when he was seven years old and all they told me was that he had been rescued from a home that had too many animals. Often rescue cats get sent to several different places in a short amount of time before they find a permanent home. That can create a lot of stress, a lot of tension and anxiety, and that can manifest in a lot of ways like digestive problems, crying and aggressiveness, hiding, biting, hitting. When I adopted Oscar, he exhibited all of the above. He was a very difficult cat to work with. I could tell that he had a loving nature underneath, but because of his history it was very hard for him to open up and relax around people. When the doorbell rang, he would run and hide. When the phone rang, he would run and hide.

My advice about choosing a cat is to select it by personality and then to make sure that the breed fits your lifestyle. I don't like cat hair so that's why I choose the hairless cats. I'm convinced that they have the best personality, too. Very playful, very loving. When I lie on the couch, he lies in the crease of my arm and he just stares up into my eyes, purring.

Rolfing benefits everyone: the animal, the owner, the other animals that are living in the house, your interaction together, and most of all their health. Cats can live a long time if they're in good health, so this is not only treating a current condition but it's also preventative. There are no harmful side effects to it, only positive benefits. Rescue animals especially benefit from Rolfing because it can really help with their traumatic history.

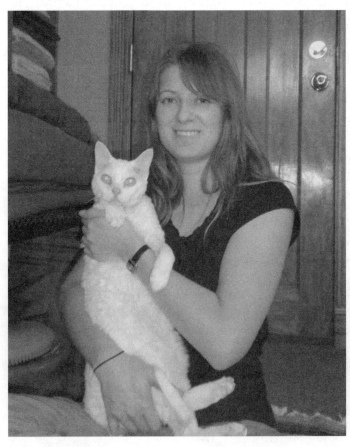

Oscar with his rescue mom, Jessica.

Resolving Emotional and Physical Trauma

An Inteview with Kathy Leffingwell about her dog, Iggy

Kathy Leffingwell: Iggy is an American Eskimo dog going on his fourth year. He belongs to my niece, Julie, but he spends time with me every week. I was getting Rolfing® Structural Integration and energy work from Briah, and during those sessions we talked about her experiences working on animals. I became interested in having Iggy's problems addressed through Rolfing as well.

This breed is usually highstrung and Iggy certainly was that. He was kind to everyone he knew, but with strangers coming to the door he couldn't settle down—he'd always yap and be in motion. It seemed like a useless waste of energy for him when he was so kind at most times.

My niece, Julie, and her then fiance adopted Iggy from the Minneapolis Humane Society. Iggy connected with Julie when they were looking for a dog and she chose him.

I think Julie's fiance had some issues with being abandoned by his mother at a young age. He was good to Iggy and took him for walks. My niece was in school full time and taking care of the house. Her fiance worked full time but he still took the time to take Iggy for out for walks. I started dog sitting in the summer of 2006 when they left for a couple of days. He enjoyed staying with me and I enjoyed him. He filled the need in my life for a dog and since Julie lived close by, we began having me take him every Wednesday to walk and play with him.

Briah Anson: Talk to me about what was happening between the two adults that affected Iggy.

KL: I believe Julie and her fiance were happy to start with. They got married the summer of 2007 and moved down to Cannon Falls. Then the marriage crumbled and they filed for divorce, Julie keeping Iggy. I don't think it was a happy home during that time. He had became abusive to Julie, and was drinking quite a bit.

I believe Iggy may have been abused as well. He had become wary of men. He likes women a lot more, finds them comforting. Julie's now ex-spouse wore a mechanic's uniform, and Iggy gets especially worked up when someone like the UPS man or mailman comes to the door. The uniform seems to get Iggy truly agitated.

Iggy had three Rolfing sessions. I had told Julie I was going to have him Rolfed, and she was fine with that. She saw the progress I was experiencing. I brought him in for the first session when I was having one of mine. Briah and I had agreed that I would have the first session and then he would have a session, but he came right up to Briah, looked directly at her and made it apparent that he wanted to be first. I was fine with that, so I brought in his blanket. He had no fear of Briah meeting her that first time, and I almost want to say he welcomed a person that could communicate to his soul. Someone who could listen in a way that I couldn't. I knew something was wrong and could sense something was unhappy with him but Briah seemed to make him feel that he finally had a voice to have it come through. He loved the session. He was a little nervous because there was noise in the hallway which made him tense up and bark.

We assured him he was safe and we would protect him and then he calmed down again and enjoyed the Rolfing session. Briah noticed that he must have been kicked pretty hard and questioned me about that. I put two and two together and assumed that the ex-husband must have done something to him during that period of unhappiness.

BA: And I would add that through his mid-body there was a lot of scar tissue. The tissues were extremely tense and he was very sensitive, almost nipping at me. It looked to me like a protective reaction.

KL: Briah suggested a homeopathic remedy at that point, so we gave him a dose. She sent some additional remedy home with me and I gave him two more doses. He is a different dog now. He is much happier and calmer with people. I continue to reassure him when he sees someone in the yard or in the neighborhood. I tell him he's okay, I'm going to protect him, the doors are locked, and he seems to be okay with it now. When someone comes whose energy does not feel right to him he still barks, but he is a changed dog. He always had happy bright eyes but now that's even more pronounced. He has settled into his body and he has none of that tension as if he was always on alert. When he sleeps, he sleeps. He can go to sleep anytime and nap during the day, whereas he used to just go to bed when Julie or I did, but he never really slept. His eyes would close but with any noise or movement, even a silent one, his eyes would flash open.

BA: It would startle him.

KL: Yeah. And now he'll just surrender to the rest he needs, especially in the last week and a half after his Rolfing session. We had two more sessions after that first one. He knew immediately when we pulled into the parking lot of the office building that we were going to see Briah. He knows her now and is excited to see her.

When I can do it, I'm going to continue on with the Rolfing for him, because I think it benefits Julie too. She has noticed that he is not so tense and it helps her. She is driven but her personality isn't anxious. Now he seems to be realizing that not being anxious is the secret to happiness.

BA: So what did you observe in the course of that second session?

KL: He wasn't worried about what was going on outside of the office this time. He knew what to expect and this session was even better. It affected him deeply into his nervous system. He just surrendered to it.

We hadn't planned to give him a third session but there was an opening after my own so we decided to do one. When I went out to get him he was looking out of the car at the office windows which he recognized. He didn't need to be convinced to come. During these second and third sessions he would roll over and be on his back which is the ultimate in trust. You could have braided his hair and he wouldn't have cared. It was bliss for him. He didn't have to be Iggy the protector, he could be Iggy . . . the recipient.

With that breed their tail is always curled up with heat coming from it—from the body to the tail. With all of his limbs and tummy open like that, you know he is happy when he can finally relax that tail. That's relaxed. And more importantly, he carried it back from the office into his own world. So I have been a very big proponent of Rolfing for anyone who needs help, and for any animal that needs a human voice to talk to about their problem.

BA: And the right *kind* of touch. I am going to add this: it was very obvious to me as the Rolfer™ that there was a lot of scar tissue through his tummy area. When he reacted in a very startled way, it showed me that he had been kicked or abused in some way. He had to always be on guard. And his not being able to sleep or rest was because his fight-or-flight response was always on. During the second and third sessions progressively, he was able to let me work deeper. He wasn't worried at all. He was almost in an altered state.

KL: Very much so, and he carried that back into his world of Julie and myself, and on his walks. When I used to meet people on our walks he would be anxious to get going, but now he just sits there waiting and looks up in the trees. He knows he'll get his walk in and he can finally enjoy other dogs. He is not so leery and I trust him now. I live in an enclosed circle neighborhood and sometimes in our early morning walks I let him off his leash. He knows I trust him to follow me but he can go explore which makes him as happy as a little kid. It gives me pride that he trusts me and I trust him.

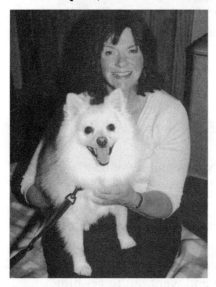

After only three sessions of my work with Iggy his fearful, anxious, and nervous way of being in the world has been transformed.

Julie has noticed that he doesn't bark, even when he comes to my house. She lets him out of the car without being on his leash, and he just runs up to the front door. But he doesn't bark. He'll wait. He is more patient. He is more patient to get food. He'll try to talk to me and Julie about what his needs are instead of pouting. He is more playful and instead of just taking the ball and me having to chase him and get it out of his mouth, he'll drop it and wait for me to toss it or he'll toss it back to me. It's nice. He's more appreciative of his life.

He's acting like a much younger dog, but more mature, instead of acting his age but immaturely, if that makes sense.

BA: Like the anxious part is gone.

KL: He doesn't need it anymore. He gets deeper love from other people and other things when he can just be himself instead of yap yap yap yap.

I think it's wonderful to adopt a pet but the unknown will always be the unknown. They've gone through a separation and that can create issues and problems. It is a wonderful thing to rescue an animal but its really wonderful to go further and give the gift of a Rolfing session. It will benefit the pet, the owner, the family, and even the neighborhood. The pet will be more connected to himself and become the best he can be. The owner is always the beneficiary of that, and the pet will know that he's really cared for. It's a wonderful bonding experience for both, and a deep appreciation of love. He can take in more of the care and the love that he's being given and give it back twicefold. It's a very small investment, and in my opinion, the road together will be easier because the ickiness is out of his body, just like a human. It's taking up space when there are better uses of his time and energy.

I had put off getting the Rolfing for myself, but I finally had to deal with the issues that were holding me back. I wanted to share my experiences only with the people that loved me and gave me support through a difficult time, which were Iggy and Julie. Julie is considering Rolfing now too. It's always the right time, when a person is ready to receive it. I've truly gone to the very soul of my body. I'm a new person. I was given the gift of awareness, and now I know what true happiness feels like. I can remember how I felt nine months ago—all the heaviness—but now there is light coming into my body all the time.

Iggy continues to only get better. He gains confidence every time he doesn't bark. He knows he's still protecting, but he has a taste of what happiness is and that he doesn't have to bark. Iggy doesn't have to be anxious anymore. He's okay being Iggy and he's okay being my niece's dog and he's okay being my part-time dog. He is a testament to what the Rolfing work can do for a human or an animal's spirit, and he's happier, truly happier.

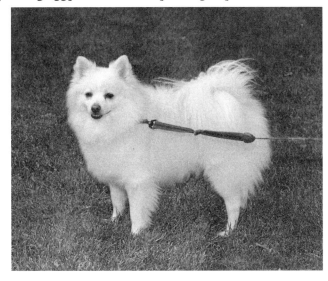

Iggy, American Eskimo dog, aligned and happy

Healing from Pet Store Trauma

An interview with Anna Dains and her daughter, Olivia,
about their guinea pigs, Eleanor, Abigail, and Rosa

Olivia Dains: We had gotten these three guinea pigs from a pet store and we think they were about a month old—they were small enough to pick up in one hand. Originally, we had only planned to get two but there were three in the cage together and we couldn't separate them because they'd been together so long. They were probably not from the same litter because they are different breeds.

Anna Dains: Eleanor was the shyest of the three guinea pigs when we bought her. In fact, she was the one that didn't come out of the little enclosure in the pet store. She was the one that was the most timid, the most frightened. Shortly after we got them, Eleanor came down with something like a cold, and she was sneezing and discharging a lot, so we were a little concerned.

Well, I think we were actually very concerned because it's often a fatal condition for guinea pigs. Any respiratory infection can be fatal and they can get really sick very quickly, something that you always treat. We hadn't taken them to the vet yet, but we just mentioned it to Briah and she offered to come and work with Eleanor.

After the First Rolfing® SI Session: Relaxed, Calm, and Thriving

OD: I thought Eleanor responded really well to her first Rolfing session. She is a very sweet natured guinea pig, but she seemed to be very calm and enjoyed it. At first she was a little tense because she didn't know who Briah was, but gradually she seemed to relax and then stretch out. When Briah put her back into the cage, she seemed to be very, very calm.

AD: So after the session, I noticed that Eleanor seemed to be relaxed to human touch a lot more. She was the most timid and the least accustomed to humans, so this changed for her. I don't know if it's possible to assess this for a guinea pig, but she was more comfortable and fluid in her body. She moved more fluidly. She seemed fuller, and she grew faster. I believe she might have been a little bit older than the other two but she did indeed grow faster than the others did.

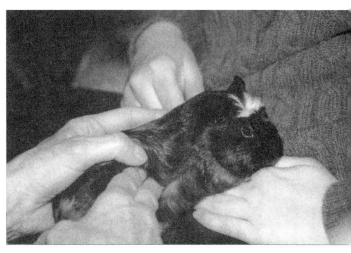

Eleanor, the guinea pig basking in all the attention.

After she came through this illness, we did go to the vet for medication, but it didn't seem to do a whole lot for her. It seemed to us that the Rolfing had been the significant turning point for her immune system. The discharge stopped very soon after those sessions, within twenty-four hours or so. She wasn't hiding in her cage as much. I'm sure part of it was also just the acclimation to humans and a new environment. We had just gotten her.

OD: When we took her to the vet she responded really well to the vet handling her, and when they put her on the table she was really curious, looking around. She didn't seem at all scared and usually when I take animals in, they're freaked out, they do not like going to the vet! This was not long after she'd had the first session. She had two sessions, and then Briah came back a week or two later. We had quarantined Eleanor from the other two guinea pigs because we were afraid she might be contagious. Not long after the second session we put her back with the other guinea pigs and she went from being the really shy one to being the dominant, the "Alpha Pig." After the second session, Eleanor became very assertive and she still is! She is the Queen Pig. She's named after Eleanor Roosevelt.

When Briah came the first time to work with Eleanor, she also Rolfed Rosa and Abigail. They weren't quite as receptive as Eleanor. I noticed that afterward Rosa and Abigail felt different. The shape of their bodies was more solid, more muscular. They also calmed down. Those two tend

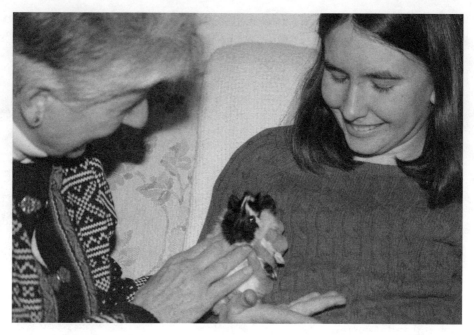

Rosa, receiving her turn while Olivia assists.

to be very fussy; if you take them out and hold them, they fuss. Part of it is because they're expecting some treat, but they just tend to complain more than Eleanor does about things.

AD: I don't know if that's breed again, too. They're more vocal. But all three of them have become quite easy to handle. They resist being picked up a little which is part of the nature of a small prey animal, but they are quite cuddly once they are picked up, particularly Eleanor. She is the most cuddly of all of them.

Movement, Athleticism, Curiosity

OD: When they had sessions again two weeks later, we saw similar results, but they felt even more muscular and we could see it in the way they walked. They were a little bit more upright– as much as a guinea pig can be that's on all fours.

AD: They had a smoother kind of movement. What I'm quite impressed with is that at well past six months old (and at six months a guinea pig is considered an adult) they are still behaving excitedly when they get their very favorite treats. They still do this movement called popcorning, where they sit on all fours and suddenly jump straight up in the air when they're excited. That's usually the movement of a very young guinea pig, but these three are able to still do that when they're excited and that's a really nice thing to see. It's really fun to see the little ones do it because they look like pieces of popcorn jumping up and down.

OD: When they're really excited and they think we're going to give them food, they'll run up to the side of their cage, put their paws on it, and look around. My guinea pig that we had several years before never did that. I never saw her popcorn, never saw her looking out with that curiosity. They also stand on their hind legs unsupported, kind of like a little trick dog. They have very good balance. I've never heard of guinea pigs doing that.

AD: They will do it unsupported as well as supported, when they're excited. As with any kind of pack animal or herd animal, there is usually one that leads the behavior, and it isn't necessarily the dominant one. It's usually Rosa who does that, and she has been the smallest although she's growing quite a bit now. She is the one who will come over first and she is the one most inclined to stand unsupported. But the other two will do it as well.

Maximizing Guinea Pig Health

AD: Another interesting thing about guinea pigs is that when they get sick, they generally don't recover. With good care, their lifespan can be eight to ten years, but the mortality rate is quite high once they have an infection. Before Olivia was born, we had a similar situation where we had several guinea pigs. My favorite guinea pig at that time got an infection, like Eleanor, but didn't make it. She did actually receive holistic treatment from a vet, but it was not Rolfing. There was no kind of bodywork done with her at all.

OD: The last guinea pig I had lived to be eight years old, but the vet said that she was one of the few. She'd never seen them live that long.

AD: With good care they should be able to do that, but so many people don't take care of them well. These girls have not been back to the vet since they've had the Rolfing, although we've thought about getting them a well-pig checkup. Very few of the holistic vets know how to deal with guinea pigs. They have a lot of dietary concerns, a lot of medications they can't take, and their immune response is really different from other animals. Guinea pigs used to be the most common lab test animal, but no longer—their systems just respond differently to medication, and their nutrition is different. They can't manufacture their own vitamin C, so they need vitamin C supplementation, like parsley or bell peppers.

OD: They can't have too much calcium, that's another big thing. My previous guinea pig ended up developing bladder stones because we gave her a ton of carrots—we didn't know carrots had so much calcium and that it was bad for them.

AD: So you can't give them too much spinach or too much carrot. But they can have leaf lettuce, grass, and timothy hay. Not alfalfa. That guinea pig was on an alfalfa diet too and that's high in calcium, which they can't metabolize well. So they're very different, for example, from a rabbit.

Social Behavior

OD: Having a single guinea pig was a really different situation from having a group. My previous guinea pig was living alone and there is a whole different mentality when they're together in a group. They're only harmonious to a degree. I think just by nature they don't always get along.

AD: I expected them to be real cuddly together but they aren't. They will each find a resting spot, so they're very independent. That is much different from our other experiences with guinea pigs, although we never brought three together at one time (except when we accidentally had babies many years ago). These girls are more bonded than the guinea pigs we had previously.

OD: When they were separated while Eleanor was quarantined, they didn't really like that.

AD: You could tell they were looking for her and missing her. When we have two of them out at night to play with them and we leave one behind, that one gets very nervous. She will get very upset, like Abigail was tonight, thrashing around. They've developed some amount of bonding.

OD: There's a bonding, but they also need their space, and they get into little squabbles sometimes. They do stand up for themselves.

AD: I would say Eleanor is dominant in a lot of ways but, for example, the others aren't afraid to steal a piece of parsley from her.

OD: They all steal food from each other.

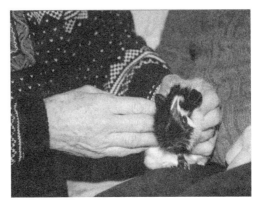

AD: There's healthy competition, and definitely Rosa, being the smallest, is not bullied. I was worried about Rosa at first that she might be bullied, but she holds her own just fine, and because she's the eager one to always get

Rosa receiving very delicate and specific work to her neck.

the first treat, sometimes she makes off with it. Abby will take her treat into the house because she has realized that nobody can get it if she does that.

OD: When they're in heat, was that any different when you had other guinea pigs? They get kind of aggressive.

AD: Yeah, they're very crabby and they do this purring. When a guinea pig makes a purring noise, it's not a sign of relaxation or affection, it's kind of a warning, and they will purr at each other when one of them is in heat. They try to mount each other, too, which is really bizarre, but not unheard of in guinea pig land. They're very grumpy girls when they're in heat.

The Rolfing Process with Small Animals: Calming, Healing Trauma and Easing Transitions

AD: I think every living creature can benefit from Rolfing. The calmness that Eleanor developed and her ease around being handled were really good for her.

OD: We don't know where they came from, or what kind of experiences they had when they were first born.

AD: Yeah, there can be a lot of shock. I really advocate getting a guinea pig from a good breeder rather than a pet store. If you're getting one from an ethical breeder you know what kind of stock you're getting, you know that the mother has received nutritional care and that it's been healthy and clean for them. We were just a little too excited and really didn't know any of the breeders in the area when we purchased these guinea pigs.

OD: There's an organization called Guinea Pig Rescue. I think it's really great if somebody is willing to take one in and take care of them, but there can be some trauma there because they could've been neglected. With our three girls, I think the Rolfing and good nutrition have been really important.

AD: Yeah, these little animals have been taken away from their mothers and then taken away from their herd and thrown into a pet store situation. They're with new little creatures, and then they're taken out of that situation into a human home. They've had a lot of disruption, separation, and transitions.

We did adopt one guinea pig that had been abused—her ears had been all chewed up so she had been abused by other guinea pigs at least. She'd been in a situation where she was dominated and that little creature never did really warm up to humans, or trust anyone. She never thrived, and she actually died shortly after childbirth. I wish we had known about Rolfing at the time and had some means to bring wholeness to that little creature.

One behavior that is very different with these guinea pigs than in our previous ones, is that the previous guinea pigs were content to sit in our laps and be petted and cuddled a little bit. These three girls we have now do not want to be held far away—they will immediately crawl up to our necks and cuddle right underneath. They're extremely affectionate. Two of them give us little kisses, and I know I've heard other owners say that, but they are the first ones we've had who have been that affectionate with us. They want to be very, very close to us.

Impatience Turns to Calm

Cindy Due, on her macaw, Loro

Loro is a six-year-old female green-winged macaw that I've had for two years. She's a large parrot for her age and breed. She's thirty-four inches from head to tail with red feathers on her head and around the eyes, white and black beak, and green, red and blue body feathers.

Loro is a real sweetheart and enjoys people, although she seems to prefer men over women. Rather than being played with or sitting on a shoulder, she likes to just be in a room with us, so she has perches throughout the house. She loves dinnertime, and eats at the table with us on her own little plate.

I don't know what her history was prior to her coming to me. I think she had a very good life but that doesn't necessarily mean that she didn't have trauma. I think she went from whoever hatched her to her first owner, then she was given to the parrot rescue, and from there she came to me. I'm her fourth home in six years, so I would assume she has had some emotional trauma—not necessarily from being abused—but going from home to home to home had to have been very hard on her. They say the average macaw is in one house for two years before it gets re-homed, and the reason for that is their tendency to scream. The owners can't take the noise. Loro's habit for two years was to start screaming at 6:00 AM after I'd gotten up to feed the dogs.

Loro had one Rolfing® session with Briah. In retrospect, it might have been better to have had Briah and Loro spend time getting to know each other first as Loro takes awhile to warm up to strangers. So Loro was acting very hesitant in the beginning, but then Briah started working on one of her wings, and it looked like Loro really got into a zone. She might have even been enjoying it. When Briah started on the other wing Loro lifted it toward Briah as if she was presenting it for treatment. I wondered how the session would have gone if Loro had met Briah a few times before being Rolfed.

During this session Loro would go from hesitancy to this interesting zone state in which I think she was releasing something out of her body. It seemed like she would go in and out of states of consciousness, and then she'd come out of it with a look that said, "Oh, what are we doing?" Then it would take a minute or two to get her relaxed again and she'd go back into another altered state. After awhile I think she'd had enough. I know that Briah hadn't gotten through her entire body, but at that point Loro let us know she was finished and wanted to go back to her cage.

When we finished the session, she spread both wings out and left them out there for about twenty seconds. She's never done that kind of presentation before. Sometimes I'll hold her up and she'll flap her wings like she is flying but she hangs onto my wrist. I thought that's what she wanted to do, so I lifted my arm up so that she could flap her wings, but she didn't. She just held her wings out to the side, as if she was showing us how big she is.

The next day she was really calm and very quiet. Then she went through three days of constant screaming. It wasn't just the chattering that parrots do, this was screaming and it was continual. Sometimes she screamed when I didn't get her out of the cage fast enough, and then she'd go to the back of the cage because she didn't want to be picked up after all. I don't know exactly what she wanted. After three days of this noisy and frustrating behavior, she was suddenly back to normal.

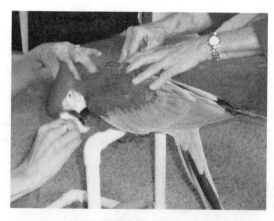

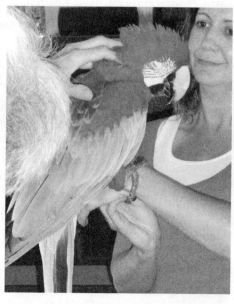

Above. *At the beginning of the first session, Cindy, Loro's owner, holds her beak in order for me to work safely.* **Right.** *Well into the session, Loro is so relaxed he could fall asleep.* **Opposite.** *At the end of the session, Loro opened her wings and kept them open with a full spread. Cindy said: "She's never done that kind of presentation before."*

She may have been releasing some old stress—perhaps from her past living situations. I've been through the Rolfing so I know it can bring up a lot of mental and emotional stuff. There were times when I'd leave Briah's office and I just wanted to go home and go to bed. I was totally exhausted and didn't want to do anything. And then there were times I'd leave there feeling energized and ready to do anything. I had about fifteen sessions and remember sometimes feeling emotional or really crabby afterward without knowing why.

One very positive thing I've noticed since Loro's Rolfing is she no longer screams at six in the morning when she sees me. She just sits and watches me. About a week after the Rolfing this morning screaming just stopped. I haven't changed my routine at all. I still get up in the morning at six o'clock, I go downstairs, I feed the dogs, and while I'm feeding the dogs, she used to scream. This has been a huge change after the Rolfing.

As far as other changes in her behavior, she seems a little more patient than she used to be. Before the Rolfing when I'd start making dinner and she'd hear the pots and pans, she used to start saying, "Step up, step up, step up!" for me to come and get her. If I didn't go to her right away she'd scream. She seems a little more patient with that now, and is content with just having me chatter at her. She also seems to be eating more.

I think the Rolfing was definitely was good for her, and I think it would be interesting for her to have another session. Birds probably need to get to know a Rolfer™ first and take it slowly. It was pretty amazing that Briah was able to do about an hour session with her even though Loro had never seen her before. It took about ten to fifteen minutes to negotiate the space, and Briah was working fairly deeply. That kind of trust was built surprisingly quickly.

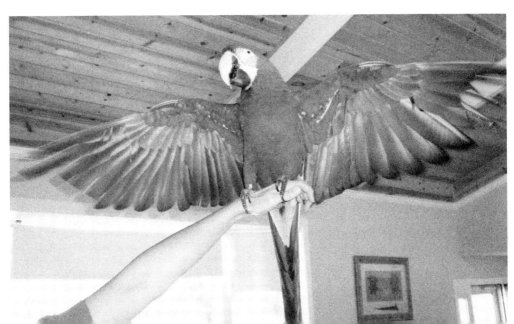

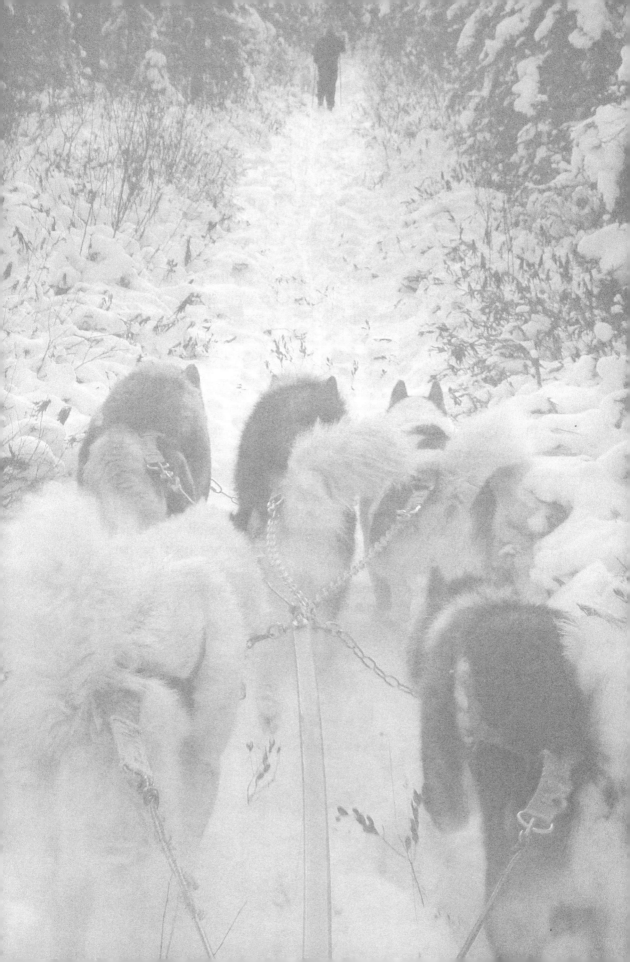

Reaching for Potential:
Animals as Athletes

▶ *Strength that has effort in it is not what you need; you need the strength that is the result of ease.*

▶ *There is a difference in energy levels of performance between the words evoke and demand.*

▶ *To me, strength is balance. Maximum strength exists in terms of muscles that are balanced.*

▶ *Robert Frost said: "You have freedom when you are easy in your harness." That is what Rolfing is about.*

DR. IDA P. ROLF, from *Ida Rolf Talks about Rolfing and Physical Reality*, Rosemary Feitis, ed., Harper Row: NY; 1978

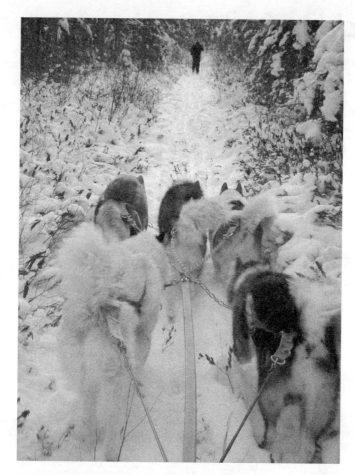

Born to pull! The sled dogs of Wintergreen.

The Sled Dogs of Wintergreen

Briah Anson, Paul Schurke, and Amy Voytilla

When I moved to Minnesota ten years ago I discovered the North Shore and the Tofte/Grand Marais area which I love. I went up to Ely one time and that's where I started hearing about the sled dogs of Wintergreen. I knew that Paul Schurke was leading sled dog trips and I had always wanted to go. It had been on my personal bucket list as one of the trips that I would very much enjoy.

Briah's Introduction to the Sled Dogs

After several years and forty sessions of working with the eagles at the National Eagle Center, I was ready for a new project. I had been wanting to meet Paul Schurke and work with his sled dogs, but I felt that I needed a connection—I didn't want Paul to say no. Then a new client came to me for healing work and said he knew Paul. He agreed to take all my materials, photographs, and articles about the work I've done with various kinds of animals and give this to Paul.

In the fall of 2009, Paul contacted me wondering if I might be willing to come up and work with some of his sled dogs, especially one by the name of Thistle. This was a ten-year-old eskimo Inuit sled dog that their vet had wanted to put down this summer. He was having a lot of pain in his hips, and his rear legs were very splayed. Paul didn't want to see Thistle put down, and shared with me that he had done a lot of water therapy with Thistle, mostly just putting him in the lake and letting him swim to see how much he could bring back his mobility. That method of rehabilitation helped Thistle by about fifty percent, but Thistle was not getting around well—he was more of a retired sled dog. Paul wanted me to come up, and wondered if I would be willing to trade a four-day trip with the sled dogs in exchange for working with Thistle and some of his other dogs.

Thistle and Rolfing® Structural Integration

I arrived at Wintergreen on a Friday evening and was scheduled to leave on Sunday. I wanted to give Thistle three very long sessions of at least an hour and a half each as a way to get the maximum amount of work into him. On Friday evening I started by taking some photographs of Thistle from both sides and from the front and back, as well as watching his gait.

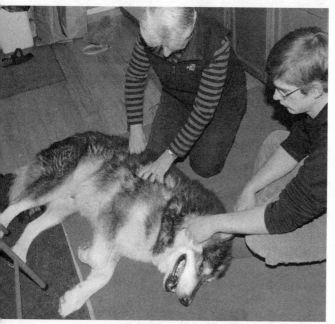

Thistle's first Rolfing® SI session as Chris Mayer assists.

Thistle had great difficulty mobilizing himself. His rear legs were very widely splayed out; they looked almost three feet apart. His top line was nearly a forty-five-degree angle, and his right leg was splayed way out as well. He was very contracted and tight, so movement was not easy for this dog.

For the next hour and a half I worked to give Thistle some ease in his structure, to release him and free up his shoulder girdle and give him some length through the spine. I finished by starting work on his hind end, which concluded the first session.

I worked again with Thistle the next morning and already his structure looked more elongated. His front legs were under him better, his stance was not as wide in the back so his legs were starting to come underneath his pelvis. I did another hour and a half session and observed that he looked like he was feeling better. His face even looked younger, as did his gait. When he walked, he was able to propel and get his rear legs coming forward underneath his body, and there was a lot more length through his structure.

On Sunday I did the last session, and this was a very interesting one. Since it was raining outside, we again did the session inside. Thistle immediately lay down and I proceeded to work a lot more deeply. I was able to rework areas where I had been before, but get in there at a deeper level. I worked to get more balance established from left to right and through the back, the torso and his hind legs.

After about a half hour of work, Thistle stood up, turned over, and presented his right hip. Now, he had never been able to do that before. In the previous two sessions, he didn't want to present that right hip. But he turned over, presented his right hip, and then turned and opened his jaw and mouth and put it completely around my hand. His teeth were not touching my hand at all, and he just looked at me. He did this two to three times, as if to say, "Okay, I want you to work there more directly, but just please be gentle with me." I almost cried. Bev, a friend who had come up with me, and I looked at each other. We couldn't believe this; it was such a touching moment.

At that point, Paul came and took Thistle from one lodge to the other one up the hill, and I saw that Thistle was running ahead and kind of pull-

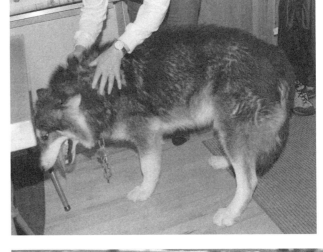

ing Paul as well, so I knew he was a lot stronger. I received a note two or three days later from Paul saying that he thought Thistle was looking a lot better, and he was waiting to hear from Thistle's owner, Amy, about what she thought when she returned.

I assured Paul that these three sessions plus some homeopathic remedies that I gave Thistle, (Rhus Tox and Arnica in some fairly strong potencies) would facilitate

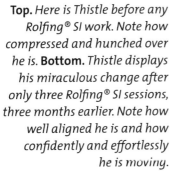

*Top. Here is Thistle before any Rolfing® SI work. Note how compressed and hunched over he is. **Bottom.** Thistle displays his miraculous change after only three Rolfing® SI sessions, three months earlier. Note how well aligned he is and how confidently and effortlessly he is moving.*

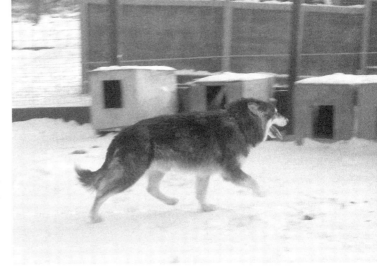

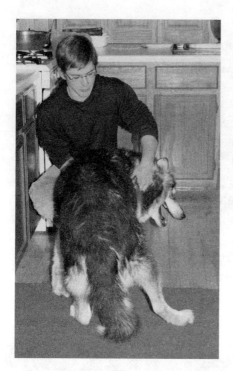 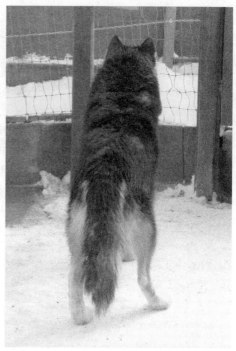

Left. *Thistle struggles to stand with the assistance of dogsled guide, Chris Mayer. Thistle's body was twisted and his rear legs so splayed that he showed very limited ability to support himself.* **Right.** *Note the dramatic change in Thistle's alignment. His legs clearly support him and his body is straight and long.*

the healing and minimize the pain and inflammation. I told Paul that in the next few weeks this work will integrate, and week by week I would expect to see Thistle healing and doing a lot better. He certainly needed more work, but I felt that the changes from that weekend's work had been fairly dramatic.

Mamo

Mamo is a very healthy, beautiful black husky. A sled dog belonging to Lisa, one of Paul's guides, Mamo had just arrived a couple of days earlier from Sweden. Lisa and her friend Chris, another one of Paul's guides, were preparing to take a four-month adventure trip across the top of Canada from one end to the other, cross-country skiing 2,200 miles in the course of four months with their team of sixteen dogs pulling all of their equipment and food. Mamo is one of these dogs, so I wanted to offer the gift of Rolfing to Mamo that evening as a way to prepare this athlete for his adventure. They had shared with me many of the challenges that they were going to be undertaking and I felt like some Rolfing work would be a very good idea. It made for a very late Friday night!

Four Sled Dog Puppies: Sweetie Pie, Storm, Bop, and Betty

The next morning I mentioned to Paul at breakfast that I had heard he had four new puppies—two brown and white ones, and two black ones, all just a month old. I told him that the most ideal time for a person or an animal to receive Rolfing SI is soon after birth. Young dogs that receive the work early will align and integrate themselves to gravity easily. They will grow in a very balanced, healthy way which will enable them to maintain a healthy structure, be tremendously strong, become great athletes, and perhaps have some of the best conformation dogs can have.

I worked for an hour on each of the four puppies. The first one was a little brown and white male who had a white bottom and we called him Sweetie Pie as he's a very, very sweet dog. Before the session I found that he felt very heavy. He was struggling against being lifted and his mus-

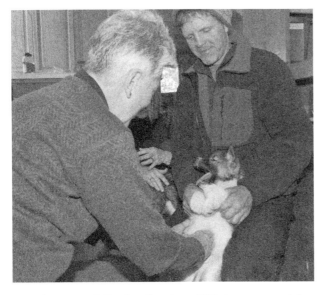
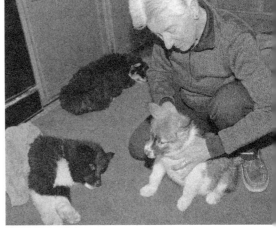
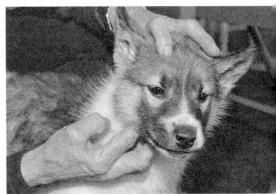

Above. *Paul Shurke, director of Wintergreen assists me while I work with Storm, a one-month-old puppy.* **Top right.** *Betty and Bop relish in the after affects of Rolfing® SI while I take a turn with Sweetie Pie.* **Bottom right.** *Sweetie Pie making the most of her turn with me.*

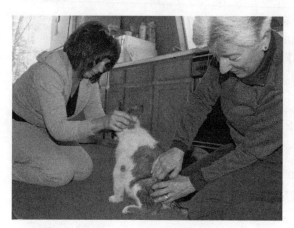

Bev Asher, a friend who accompanied me to Wintergreen for a weekend of work on sled dogs, assists me in my work with Storm.

cles seemed to stiffen. I could see that he was very compressed and his hips felt very tight. After the session he was soft everywhere and very loose. He wasn't fighting being picked up, and he felt very balanced. Lisa was there assisting me and she could also feel the changes. He looked very, very balanced.

The next puppy I worked with we named Storm after a similar dog my friend, Bev, had known. This was a second dog from the same litter, standing about a foot tall, a couple feet long, and about a foot wide, so he was already pretty hefty. It was a similar case to Sweetie Pie—different patterns in their shoulders and hip girdles, but basically the same kind of thing: freeing up the hip/shoulder, freeing up the torso, getting the legs organized and getting the hips mobilized so that their alignment would improve and be able to grow unencumbered. After the session Lisa held the puppy up and she said it just felt totally balanced.

Paul had asked me, "Why do this with a young healthy pup?" I explained that all the problems you see in the adult dog were there in the young pup. Just like in the baby, the same patterns that are in the baby or in the child, you later see in the adult at age forty or fifty or sixty, just a little bit more compressed, more hammered in. That's why it's so important to free everything up and align the structure. It affects the growth plates and the development of healthy structural relationships between all the anatomical parts. The state of the structure impacts the development of the organs and the function of how those dogs will work.

The birth process also plays a part in how the puppy's body will be after birth. These two dogs from the same litter had different issues going on, and I'm sure it had a lot to do with how they grew inside the womb. A mother dog has a large litter and there are a lot of growing puppies in a small space. Some have little room and some have more room, and they're growing in there for a number of months. These patterns can become embedded in the structure of each dog before they are even born. Each dog is developing from his own individual blueprint. Rolfing SI is a way to intervene in the evolving structure and neuromuscular development so that that blueprint can unfold into its highest potential.

Next were two black puppies that were also a month old. The first was Bop, a male with white tipped ears and white on the muzzle. Before the session Bop was very docile, and he virtually slept during the Rolfing session. He was just very calm and I was able to go very deeply into his body and do a lot of work. Paul was there at the time and had checked his range of motion in his front legs and shoulders, and he reported that the range of motion of the front legs and shoulders was greater after the Rolfing session. The other puppy was Betty, a female, and Paul had felt some lumps in the shoulder girdle before the Rolfing session. After about fifteen minutes of work, I had Paul examine the area where I had been working around the shoulder girdle and he reported that the range of motion was greater and the lumps were gone. The dog was a lot looser and more relaxed.

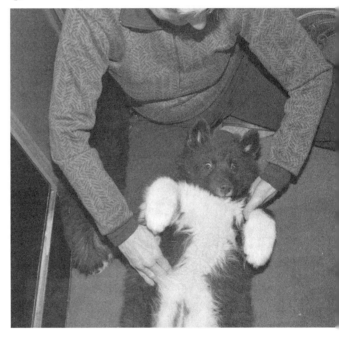

Betty making the most of her turn with me.

Three Mature Sled Dogs: Goofy (Regal), Jenz, and Heinzie

That Saturday afternoon I worked with three mature sled dogs that were all having structural issues. They were older dogs, around ten years of age. The first one that I worked with had been named Goofy officially, but my friend Bev and I renamed him Regal. He was a big white dog who looked very regal, and he had an attitude. We were outside and each of the three dogs were secured to a cable about eight feet apart. Regal was not too happy about the work. I started by just barely working with his shoulder girdle and he growled in a very menacing way, and then bared his teeth. Every now and then Paul walked by because he was involved in some project, and I mentioned to Paul that I was a little bit concerned about this level of growling that felt very aggressive. Paul said, "Oh, don't worry about it, he's just growling about the other dogs," but I knew the other dogs were minding their own business and it felt very much related to the work. So I was not too sure how this was going to go with Regal.

After trying to negotiate with him, trying him to get him to lie down or sit, which he didn't want to do, I just decided to say to Regal straight out, "If you don't lie down in the next three seconds, I guess I'll have to go work on the next dog." Immediately, that dog starting digging a little shallow hole. He dug it out and turned around and lay down. I worked away on his front end for a while and he started to get agitated again as I worked on his hips. He then got up and moved around, so I said again, "Well, I guess if you don't want to lie down, I might have to work on the other dog." Again, he did the same thing, so it was clear that we had an understanding. I was able to work on him for more than an hour, and by the end of the session he looked a lot better. He moved about eight feet away and just lay down looking very, very content.

The next dog I worked with was Jenz who had been worked hard over the years and was pretty bound up. He had observed the interaction that I had had with Regal and he was immediately very compliant, allowing me to work quite deeply. So that session went without any event and he looked better.

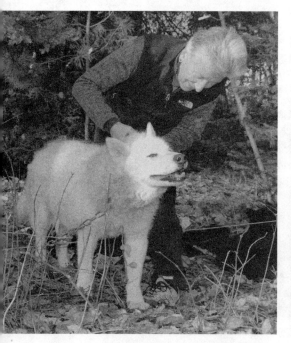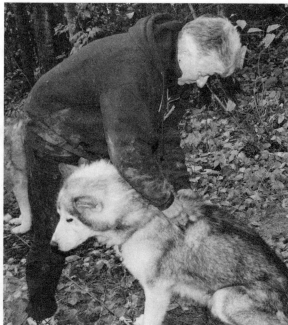

Left. *Goofy, a challenging spirit, finally accepting the work.* **Right.** *Jenz, being released from all that pulling.*

Then I moved on; it was getting closer to dark. Heinzie was also extremely cooperative. I think that it was helpful having the interactions that I did with Regal because the other dogs just lined up perfectly and I was able to get a lot of work done very quickly.

The next day I gave Regal his second session. It was raining as it was getting close to winter, so we went inside a cabin and Regal immediately lay down. There was no problem. He even turned and presented that right hip and I worked for well over an hour. My assistant, Bev, kept just talking to him, and this dog had his eyes closed and he looked like he was smiling. Paul came and got Regal, and I saw Regal really pull Paul up the hill, so I feel the dogs who were in the worst shape, Thistle and Regal, were left feeling a lot better.

I am really quite excited about continuing my relationship with Wintergreen. They have about ninety dogs, and I'm sure they can all use the work. Paul is doing a wonderful thing providing these dogsled trips for people. People who go there learn to appreciate the animals and the boundary water canoe environment of Ely. It's an exquisite area and a wonderful journey for people to take. I feel that anything I can do to evoke the health, longevity, and the wellbeing of these dogs is well worth doing.

Paul Schurke Reflects on His Sled Dogs and Briah's Visit to Ely

We like to think of these dogs as Olympic athletes because pound for pound they burn up more calories than just about any organism I'm aware of. They live to pull, they love to pull, and they're incredibly hardworking animals. We've wondered what kind of a toll their love for pulling takes on them physically, and we've noticed that in addition to loving to pull, they also love to be handled.

They're extraordinarily affectionate and sociable, but I think their solicitation of handling also has something to do with just the pleasure that they find in being handled by people. Not just a pat on the head, but actually a bit of a rubdown feels good to them. They really perk up when we start working, kneading our fingers into their backs or their shoulders. So we wondered if something more substantial along those lines might be useful to ensure their health and wellbeing—to have more significant manipulation done by someone who is in the know about what sort of manipulation can be most effective for working animals.

Then much to our astonishment, good friends here in Ely had passed along information about just the person who is an expert in that par-

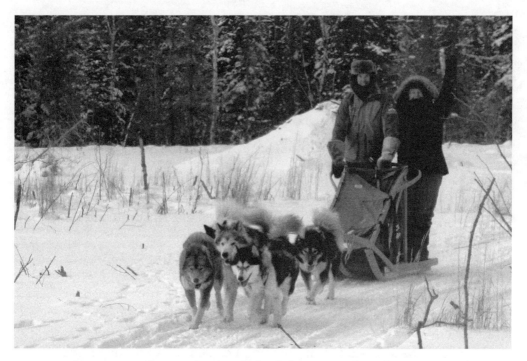

Taking timeout from work to mush the sled dogs on a three-day trip in Northern Minnesota.

ticular area, Briah Anson. She has specialized and carved out quite a unique niche for herself in applying Rolfing® Structural Integration to animals of all kinds, wild and domestic. We wanted to see whether those techniques would apply beneficially to working animals as well—draft animals, or more specifically, draft canines. So we seized the moment and brought Briah up here to find out what this Rolfing work was all about and how it might apply to our working animals, and she was kind enough to oblige us in that.

Over the last couple of months we've learned a lot about Rolfing SI and seen it applied to some of our dogs. We've had an opportunity to witness the benefits that they appear to be gaining from that care.

Exhibit A is a dog named Thistle. Our connection with Briah was particularly timely in that regard, because just prior to learning about Briah and her services in September, 2009, our beloved sled dog, Thistle, developed a nerve disorder where his hips just up and gave out on him. He wasn't able to maintain his stance anymore. Conventional veterinary care didn't seem to offer him many options.

Thistle belongs to one of our staff, Amy Voytilla, so I'm a little out of the loop on exactly what transpired when Thistle's mishap occurred. At some point he was no longer able to get up, and it was apparent that he had no sensation or control of his hindquarters and was only able to drag himself around on his front legs. Amy had brought him into the vet and after a couple of sessions, they determined that there was little hope and the prognosis wasn't good. With the paralysis in his hips, he was likely to soon become incontinent and then would suffer an agonizing demise with bowel and bladder infections. Understandably, the recommendation was to put him down; that was the most humane thing to do rather than oblige him to undergo the discomfort of a long anguishing demise.

But given our affection for Amy and her Thistle, and particularly Amy's affection for Thistle, Amy was not ready to follow the vet's suggestion. So Thistle came home here, and dragged himself around as we puzzled about what we might try on our own.

Realizing that the problem was a lack of control of his hindquarters, we assumed it had to be a pinched nerve. We came up with a little ad hoc technique as a last ditch effort to see if we could get some freedom of movement in his spine in hopes that the nerve would reconnect, which was a layman's version of water therapy. We put a life jacket on Thistle, floated him out on our beach here, and oddly enough it appeared to help because he clearly gained some muscle function in his hips again. That gave us hope that maybe it wasn't time to say good-bye to him.

Thistle lived on with the daily doses of water therapy, paddling around on the beach with a life jacket holding up his hindquarters, and he gained increasing use of his rear legs. It was apparent that there was some healing going on but he had a long way to go. The water therapy bought us some time to try something more significant, and something more significant happened along when Briah Anson came up here and spent a weekend doing Rolfing sessions with him. It was very effective in furthering his healing process and allowed him to gain additional use and control of his hips.

The nerve damage, or whatever had caused this problem, gave him a side slip. Occasionally he would have a misfire in his nerves and his legs would fall out from under him. He'd have to struggle to get back up again. When he was able to walk the weight of his torso pulled his hips sideways. But now that has straightened up, and while he may still occasionally have a misfire in the nerves, it is nothing that is significantly noticeable. In fact, for someone seeing Thistle for the first time they would assume that he is as happy and healthy as any dog here. He has made a remarkable recovery, and his gait is true and straight again, presumably a reflection of enhanced spinal alignment that allows him to hold his back and hips properly. This has been very encouraging.

Thistle now is back to his usual old self. He may never be a full bore pulling dog again but he is also of an age where he probably would have been retiring soon regardless. He is clearly happy and relatively healthy and has sufficient use of his hindquarters and his legs now to carry on as he always had down in the kennelry, running around in an open pen with other dogs. Bowel and bladder functions are just fine and all systems are go, so Thistle is a wonderful success story of a dog for whom there was otherwise little hope. The Rolfing process appears to have given us the edge we needed to ensure that he could carry on a meaningful life.

Goofy is another dog that we had Rolfed. Despite his prosaic name, Goofy is the real thing. He is a Greenlandic Inuit dog from the northern-most village in Greenland. He came to us from an Inuit family who obviously had a sense of humor to give the dog a name like that.

Goofy had experienced the same kind of life as most Arctic dogs where they live in a very extreme environment and work very hard. Goofy was on a polar bear hunting team and if Goofy could tell stories, I'm sure he would have a bestselling book in the works by now given the experiences that he has had.

But he was given to us when he was a few years old, young enough to still be full of vim and vigor, but his life in Greenland had taken its toll. The dogs in the Arctic age quite early. Our dogs here at Wintergreen have a pulling life that extends from about eight months when we first put them to harness, to ten or twelve years of age. Compared with other working animals, our dogs have a fairly cushy life here at Wintergreen— lots of love and affection, good food and good fun. Life is a little more serious in the high Arctic and for those dogs, their pulling career might extend from eight months of age until four to six years, which is getting to be an old dog in the Arctic. So Goofy was well on his way toward his retirement years, as young as he was, given the rigors of Arctic life.

Since he came here and life is a little easier for him, his pulling career has been extended many years. We brought him here in 2001, and Goofy is still pulling and living a long ripe life. But the elements had taken their toll, and while the situation with his hips and back were nothing like Thistle's yet, it was apparent that he had sustained significant wear and tear on his spinal alignment and hindquarters. We had Briah work with Goofy to see if we could put a little spunk back in him as well, and I think we've seen similar benefits.

We did two sessions, not actually looking for any miracle cure. I had anticipated that Goofy would be retired this year, and would just hang out in the retirement pen, running around with the other retired dogs. But for most of these dogs, because their whole world is built around pulling, I think retirement isn't as rosy as it sounds to us. They get quite anxious when they see the other dogs being harnessed to go out for the day and they're stuck in the pen. As nice as it might be to race around in an open pen, they would still rather be doing the thing that they've done all their life, which is pulling a sled. So we're pleased now that Goofy appears to have at least another good season in him, to do what he enjoys most, being down there ready to get harnessed and go out on trail. The Rolfing sessions seem to have bought him some time to extend his pulling career and maintain a meaningful existence in that way.

The positive impact from physical manipulation through the Rolfing sessions with Briah has had interesting behavioral consequences in that Goofy now seems to quite enjoy being handled.

Briah had mentioned to me when she was working with Goofy that he was growling in an aggressive way. Lyn Ann had told her that Goofy didn't like to be handled or touched, and Briah wondered if that was just because of the pain he was in. I think one of the things that comes with the territory with a dog that you bring down from the high Arctic is that in the Arctic the dogs are all business. They don't get lots of cuddling and love and affection from people like they do here. They're not beaten or abused by their Inuit masters, but they're also afforded little affection or attention. It's strictly a working relationship and that works well for life in the Arctic.

Consequently, the dogs we brought down from the Arctic are noticeably less solicitous of affection than the dogs that are raised here at Wintergreen. People who see the dogs we brought directly from the Arctic compare them with their own dogs and assume they are a completely different breed of dog because of the behavioral differences. But it's strictly a result of how they were brought up.

Goofy maintained that reticence regarding handling and affection during all the years he's been here at Wintergreen. He was approachable and personable but wasn't out there gunning to be petted every time somebody walked by like most of the other dogs are. The positive impact from physical manipulation through the Rolfing sessions with Briah has had interesting behavioral consequences in that Goofy now seems to quite enjoy being handled. He realizes that it's a good thing, that it feels good and it's good for him. He's noticeably more open and receptive to being petted and handled than he had been before. So that will make him a more popular animal in the kennel. Now that he is anxious to have human handling, more people are likely to oblige him in that.

I now have the opportunity to see the benefits of manipulation across the entire span of a sled dog's life. We had a litter of puppies here that Briah did sessions with when they were only a few weeks old. I will be interested to see how their performance compares with their older colleagues when those puppies reach pulling age.

It's an industry standard that pulling dogs are ready for harness when they're eight months old. By tradition, it's understood that their musculature and skeletal structure is sufficiently established by eight months that they can be trained in harness without stunting their growth, hence the rationale for that time frame in training them.

These puppies that Briah worked on in March of this year will be old enough to begin pulling right before the end of our season. They'll have a chance to pull in harness and be ready to go full bore next year. We can then compare how their harness training and development as pulling dogs progresses with that of previous litters who've come to harness age by March. I also want to see if they are less likely to sustain exhaustion from the long days in harness.

Just before Briah started manipulating each puppy, I would pick them up and handle them myself, noticing how they felt. Lumpy stiffness would probably characterize what I observed prior to their Rolfing sessions, and I assumed that would lead to misalignments in their joints as they grow that would be detrimental to their ability to work as pulling dogs. In terms of the puppies' alignment and movement patterns in the three months since, it's hard for me to gauge. It's impossible to know how they would have looked at this point without the Rolfing work. But I think that with over thirty years experience I will be able to observe any differences in how quickly they achieve full capacity as pulling dogs, versus dogs in the past that didn't benefit from this work.

I think there is a collateral benefit to Briah's visit for us here at Wintergreen. None of us are Rolfers™ nor would we pretend to be, but it certainly encouraged us to spend more time just simply handling our dogs. They obviously enjoy and appreciate that. They benefit from it when it's applied in a therapeutic manner, but I'm sure they benefit from it mentally when they're handled just for fun. One of the residual benefits of having had Briah up here and observing her skills is that I think we are all more encouraged as a crew to spend more time handling the dogs. Whether we are benefiting them physiologically I don't know, but I know they are benefiting psychologically. The ones that have had Rolfing sessions certainly are more inclined to solicit handling and enjoy being handled because they've felt the benefits of it, and are clearly aware that it's a good thing for them.

Amy Voytilla Talks about Her Work with Wintergreen, and Thistle

I have been a guide at Wintergreen for four years. People come for dog-sledding vacations varying from half-day trips to camping trips that can be week-long experiences. People are the mushers, so the participants are standing on the back of the sled and they learn how to not just give the dogs commands, but they're also very hands-on with harnessing the dogs and feeding them. I ski either in front of the teams or toward the back of a train of sleds, and guide people through the boundary waters area in the winter woods near Ely, Minnesota.

Thistle's troubles started this past summer when I came home from work and I saw Thistle walking around in a funny manner in the dog yard. He continued to decline over the following twenty-four hours. I have no idea what happened to him but it seemed like something was seriously wrong with his back and he gradually lost feeling in his back legs. At that point I was very scared and took him to the vet in Ely. Thistle was seven years old, which is getting close to retirement for a sled dog, but I was still expecting him to have quite a few more years.

The options the vet gave us were either surgery or steroids for a period of time to see if they could bring down swelling in whatever was pinched in his back. We took the steroid option and the vet told us that if he did not get feeling back in his legs within forty-eight hours then we should consider putting him down. Thistle stayed at the clinic for that time period and did not improve. I wanted to give Thistle a good last twenty-four hours so I brought him to Wintergreen where he was comfortable and familiar. If need be, we could put him down out here.

Paul helped me find a comfortable spot for Thistle. We settled on the dock near the lake where there was a nice breeze. This was in the middle of summer, so it was a good spot without any bugs. As Paul and I carried

Thistle to this spot (he weighs close to a hundred pounds), Paul had the idea that we might try having him swim which is part of rehabilitative therapy for people with spinal injuries. We strapped a life jacket around his middle and put him in the water. Thistle was freaked out by the experience at first. He paddled vigorously with his front two legs but after being in the water for just two or three minutes, we saw a little flutter, a little motion with one of his back legs. That was enough hope to keep going and see what happened with him.

Sure enough, throughout the next couple of days he went from moving his legs more with swimming, to actually supporting himself and sort of scooting around. Then over the course of a week he was actually standing again. That recovery in and of itself was astounding. He still had this uneven walk. He almost looked like he was drunk as he was walking—sort of a swagger in his back legs and he would lose his balance periodically. That's where the Rolfing work made a big difference.

Briah came up the first week of October when I had just left. She gave Thistle three sessions, but I didn't see him again until I returned at the beginning of December. Thistle was walking at a natural pace, either at a walk or a fast trot. He looked very coordinated and I didn't notice any splaying of his legs or any of that awkwardness. When he gets excited and moves quickly he can still lose balance in one leg and that throws him off for a second, but then he starts moving again. It is remarkable how big of a difference Rolfing has made. His top line seems pretty straight now whereas it was at a forty-five-degree angle, and his rear legs are now under him.

With the start of the dog sledding season, all of the dogs get very excited, raring to go, and he's right in there with them, wanting to go. He's as chipper as he's ever been at the start of the season. I have let him out in the past few days and he trots around looking important.

We took a half-day trip out the other day, traveling with a couple teams of dogs, and I was surprised when Thistle decided to follow us. He actually got in front of me where I was skiing in front of the teams. We were out about three hours and covered two or three miles through a lot of snow. We went downhill onto a frozen lake where the snow span and traction can be an issue, and then through a boggy area with uneven ground. I was watching him go through this terrain, and I'd see one of his feet go lower than another, but he always regained his balance. He was pretty tired by the end of the day, but he was ready to go again the next and his gait was still good.

I'm so glad we had the opportunity to get the Rolfing work for him. None of the traditional options were good ones—either put him down, or do a surgery that was terribly invasive, minimally successful, with a recovery that required keeping him crated for months. I felt so fortunate that Paul thought of the swimming therapy that brought back the use of his legs, and then he was able to get the Rolfing sessions that brought him completely back on track. It wasn't invasive or scary for him, and it sounded like he enjoyed the sessions.

The Sled Dogs of Wintergreen

These dogs are a fascinating breed with interesting and unusual lives. I have included information, with permission, from Paul Schurke's website, www.dogsledding.com, so that you can learn more about them.

Paul has about ninety purebred Canadian Eskimo dogs, which are the centerpiece and key staff members of Wintergreen. This breed, the original sled dog of the high Arctic, (and now commonly referred by the more politically correct name: Canadian Inuit Dog), is considered to be the "Sherman Tank" of the mushing world. The breed evolved with the Arctic cultures which employed them as draft animals. These dogs absolutely live to pull. In fact, the pulling instinct is so strong that they need little training. We first harness our dogs at about eight months of age, team them up alongside a seasoned veteran for training, and within minutes they dig their feet in and their line goes taut as that intense pulling instinct clicks on like a light. Their pulling career extends ten to twelve years and then they retire to a condominium cooperative near Naples, Florida. (Just kidding! Actually, they get the run of the place at Wintergreen.)

The Rich History of the Wintergreen Dogs
Canadian Inuit dogs were the mainstay of Arctic transport for thousands of years. But when the snowmobiling frenzy swept the Arctic in the late sixties, the dogs fell into disuse and the breed all but disappeared. Now, however, the breed is making a comeback in Greenland and the eastern Arctic as villagers have taken a renewed interest in this central element of their cultural heritage. Because of their strength and ability to thrive in extreme conditions, Canadian Inuit dogs were selected to power the first expeditions to reach the North Pole (Robert Peary in 1909) and the South Pole (Roald Amundson in 1911). In fact, they have been employed

on virtually all nonmechanized polar expeditions since, including the six North Pole expeditions that Wintergreen has been involved with.

Wintergreen's breed stock were secured from four main sources. We purchased our first team of Inuit dogs from an Inuit hunter on the island of Igloolik (near the mouth of Hudson Bay). Then, in 1992, we were selected by the Australian government as their kennel of choice to provide a new home for the last team of working dogs still in use at an Antarctic research station. Those dogs, which originated from Inuit dogs brought to Antarctica over fifty years ago, have fit in fine with our kennel. The transition was the subject of an award-winning National Geographic film called "The Last Husky." In 1993, we received a team of Inuit dogs from a family in Baffin Island. Most recently, we've brought a dozen Inuit dogs back with us from our trips with the Polar Eskimos of northern Greenland.

The Working Dogs of Winter

Canadian Inuit Dogs are one of four main working breeds of the far north, which also includes the Siberian Husky, the Malamute and the Samoyed. The Siberian Husky and their mixed breed cousins (commonly called Alaskan Huskies) are the fastest and thus the breed of choice for racers, though they range only forty to sixty pounds in size. The Samoyed breed was developed as a sled dog by the Samoyed people of the Russian arctic. But during the last century, European and American dog lovers were more attracted by the breed's beautiful white coat and today Samoyeds are more commonly found in the pet show circuit than in harness.

Malamutes are the largest of the pulling dogs and typically weigh more than a hundred pounds. They were developed by the Malamute people of western Alaska (a culture that no longer exists) and became famous for pulling the Forty-Niners and their supplies over the Dawson Trail during the Alaskan Gold Rush. They remain popular today as family pets and pulling dogs. But because their sheer size makes them unwieldy for novice mushers to handle, they are rarely used for recreational dog-sled programs.

Averaging eighty pounds, the Canadian Eskimo Dog falls between the Malamute and Husky in size. That means they've got the beef and build for back country travel but can still be comfortably handled by most beginners. Most of them are extremely personable. Like their cousins, the Arctic wolves, they have extremely strong pack instincts. The pack hierarchy is always changing. Therefore some of them will not run to-gether without sparring over dominance. Reading these changes in the pack hierarchy and pairing the dogs up appropriately is part of the chal-lenge and mystery of working with these amazing animals. In 1996, the Discovery Channel produced a documentary on the Inuit dog in which Wintergreen's dogs are prominently featured.

Our Dogs: Olympic Athletes with Lots of Personality
At Wintergreen our ninety Canadian Inuit Dogs comprise the largest ken-nel of this breed in the United States. People often ask: "how do you tell of your dogs apart?" That's easy because each has such a distinct person-ality. Our guests are always surprised how distinct and unique each dog is. As we say here at Wintergreen, working with a team of six dogs is like working with a team of six people. Each has his or her own needs and abilities. They'll work together and get the job done but maximizing their performance requires good leadership. That's what mushing is all about. You basically become the coach of a team of Olympic-caliber athletes.

And they truly are athletes. An Inuit dog will pull at least twice its weight in payload at a pace of five to six miles per hour for hours at a time. Their thick double coats and tough demeanor allow them to thrive in extreme conditions. In fact, the colder it is, the harder they pull. They're accustomed to eating snow for moisture and, when night comes, they curl into a ball, wrap their tails over their noses, settle into the snow and sleep soundly. Come daybreak, they all pop up with the slightest hint around camp that sleds are being loaded and anxiously paw the air, seeking to be the first to be harnessed. Wintergreen guests are continuously amazed at how hard these dogs work and how much they love it.

And dogs that love to pull are lucky to be at Wintergreen because they enjoy a very long pulling season. We begin cart training in October when the weather cools. By late November we've got sufficient ice and snow to switch to sleds. And then they're in use at least five days a week during our program season in the Ely area from December through March. Come April and May, many of the dogs are used for our Wintergreen West pro-grams near Yellowstone and our expeditions to Hudson Bay, Ellesmere Island and the North Pole. That means there's only four months (June-September) of "poor sledding'" for Wintergreen dogs.

Sled Dogs One Year Later

An Update from Paul Schurke, October 16, 2010

About a year ago Briah was here and did Rolfing® sessions on a number of our sled dogs: four of the puppies, three sessions with Thistle, two with Goofy, and one each with Heinz and Jenz.

Of course, Thistle is the cover story dog. He truly is a remarkable story in that he was a dog whose hips had locked up and to all appearances had become paralyzed from the lower part of his spinal column back, with no use of his hindquarters. After medication and visits to the vet, the prognosis was not good, and they had suggested it might be time to say a sad good-bye to Thistle. But he was too dearly loved for that and his dear friend, Amy, was determined to leave no stone unturned and try other options. We tried a little ad hoc hydrotherapy with Thistle that is related in the preceding story about the sled dogs.

Briah arrived when Thistle was showing some promise, and following his Rolfing sessions, he took a quantum leap forward and showed considerable additional movement, and has been his happy lovable self ever since. Given his age, we had no expectation of him becoming a full-bore sled dog. He is enjoying a well-earned retirement, but he is enjoying it with far greater freedom of movement now than he certainly would have otherwise. So we are all very happy that Thistle is still with us and that Amy still has that friend in her life. Thistle is quite clearly enjoying his ability to run around the woods as he's always done.

In fact, there is more to the story. Occasionally throughout this last season, because he had shown such remarkable recovery, there were at least a couple of half-days where he begged and begged when the teams were being harnessed to join the fun. Amy did slip him in a harness, so he got out for a half day from time to time, to be part of a pack once more. I believe he was cut loose in the afternoons so we wouldn't unduly stress his aging bones and joints, but it was certainly a minor canine miracle to see Thistle in harness again. No one here would have ever anticipated that, considering how far he'd come from the sad stretch of time when he had no use of his hindquarters whatsoever.

Free to roam, a loving companion, and living the kind of golden years that all of us hope our sled dogs will enjoy, because they live to pull, and they pull until they're age nine, ten, eleven. Then most of them, as is the case here at Wintergreen, enjoy winding down for a few years in an open pen. They goof around together, and they'll live to be twelve, thirteen, fourteen. Our oldest was a beloved lead dog named Snow White who lived to be fifteen.

We consistently observe that the dogs that enjoyed Rolfing sessions have exceeded our expectations regarding their performance, whether they're young dogs, pups, or the older dogs. Across the board, from our poster child Thistle, to our young up-and-comer Betty, in comparison with others of their age and rank, they excel.

Briah did a couple major sessions on Goofy. Goofy was an older dog and because we had brought him from Greenland, we are not exactly sure of his lineage. He appeared to have some congenital hip issues. We rarely see that in this breed. He is a Canadian Inuit dog, the original working dog of the high Arctic, and the one and only indigenous domesticated canine of North America—a pure, but in many ways primitive, breed. Of course in this context, primitive is a plus because it also means that they're not burdened by the congenital defects that accompany hybrid dogs, and the overbreeding that does a terrible disservice to the health and vitality of a dog. Fortunately, the Canadian Inuit dog, being an ancient breed, is free from those defects, especially hip dysplasia. We never see this in our dogs but Goofy showed some signs of it.

In Greenland it's a free-for-all with breeding programs because the Inuit dogs often just run free among the villages along with other breeds, so inbreeding is a distinct possibility. He may well have had some inbreeding that led to congenital hip dysplasia, or at least some minor indications of that. So he had that strike against him in attempting to work his way into old age as a pulling dog, but I think some manipulation and Rolfing therapy assisted him in his ability to carry on. He pulled all through the winter last year, and he has since passed away, but he did go out with his boots on, as we all hope to do.

Briah did long sessions on Heinzie and Jenz, who rank among the oldest dogs in the kennel. Typically dogs of their age are candidates for an occasional day in harness, maybe a half day, but largely they have settled into retirement. However, both Heinzie and Jenz went full steam last season and they appear to be at full vim and vigor at the end of this summer and early fall. All the indications are that they will be pulling at least part time, maybe full time, and maybe the whole season this year as well. It's a little hard to gauge until we get them out on the early season trips and find out if they can go the distance for a full day, or maybe it will end up that they are happier just doing half a day. But we do know these dogs love to pull and live to pull, and if we can extend their pulling career and extend their sense of usefulness and activity, it certainly enhances their quality of life. So if the Rolfing has helped extend their pulling career for another winter or two, then it will certainly be a credit to the art of Rolfing and a service to the well-being of these animals.

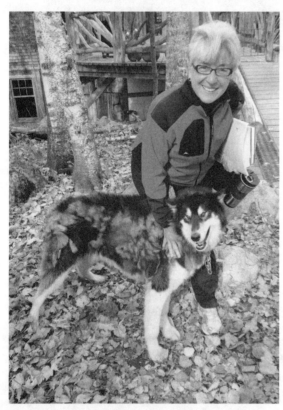

Feeling the restorative power of Rolfing® SI, Moe snuggles into me to say his goodbyes as I leave Wintergreen.

A year ago in October there were four new pups who received Rolfing sessions from Briah. Unfortunately, a mishap befell that litter when a couple of them succumbed to canine parvovirus. This is a devastating viral infection that young dogs are highly prone to. It's just luck of the draw—it comes sweeping through kennels from time to time, and we got hit for the first time in years with a run of parvovirus last season. We lost a couple pups but their sister, Betty, survived and is a spirited, rambunctious, some might even say overly energetic young female, bouncing off the walls of that kennel. In fact, she is so spirited that she has spent the summer in an open pen with a bunch of adult dogs. Normally, we keep the younger dogs separated so they can sort out their own pecking order among dogs of similar age rank, but Betty is an unusually exuberant dog. She seems to hold her own just fine with the adults she is bouncing around with in this kennel where she has been all summer. She did a little pulling last season. We start these dogs in pulling when they are eight months of age. She had neared that just at the end of the snow season last year, so I had a chance to get a little harness training going, but she is now close to being fully grown. They don't achieve full physical maturity until they are around eighteen months. She is close to that now, and given all her energy and vigor, I'm sure she'll be one of the young all-stars this season in the kennel.

We consistently observe that the dogs that enjoyed Rolfing sessions have exceeded our expectations regarding their performance, whether they're young dogs, pups, or the older dogs. Across the board, from our poster child Thistle, to our young up-and-comer Betty, in comparison with others of their age and rank, they excel. They certainly exhibited that last season, and we expect the same this season, so it appears that the benefits were significant.

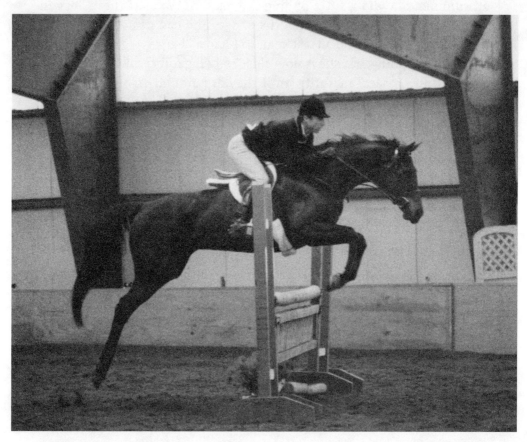

Horse and rider jumping beautifully through space. Fred Kahn, horse trainer and equestrian. Photo courtesy of Fred Kahn.

The Horse and the Rider Connect

Fred Kahn, on his horses, Petey and House

I had the Rolfing® series several years ago in Seattle, then again in Colorado. I met Briah in Kansas City five or six years ago and was interested to see how her technique would compare to those of the other Rolfers™. My first, a male Rolfer, was very powerful and made some powerful changes in me. The second Rolfer was much more subtle and into fine tuning. She was more of a detail Rolfer, and my life was also becoming more detailed and more organized. Briah approaches Rolfing from a spiritual viewpoint and makes me feel and think about the bigger picture. She hits a level of consciousness that makes me think of more important things than my next appointment at work.

Fred's Rolfing Experience

Now the question was, how did I get into Rolfing originally? As a horse trainer, I encountered many physical problems. Case in point: it is important when you are on a horse to have a straight line from shoulders to hip joint to ankle. I always seemed to have my feet out in front which caused me to roll onto my tailbone behind the horse's motion and be unable to pull my leg back. I thought, "Wow, I need some real help in changing the way I sit." I looked into lots of things. One was Feldenkrais® work which was wonderful, but slow. It works well with Rolfing, but it wasn't enough. It was subtle but I wasn't getting results. As I was looking into other things, I kept running into Rolfing but was afraid of it because I had heard it was painful.

Finally I decided to look in the phone book and found this guy. I scheduled an appointment and after the first session, knew Rolfing was for me. It did a lot more than get my leg right under the horse. It changed my position and sense of timing. I was more relaxed and could move with the horse. It changed my teaching also because I was able to recognize different movement blocks other people had. I couldn't Rolf them, but I could understand their limits and help them find a way around a particular block.

My own range of motion became so much better and freer. I used to have a closed upper body and shallow breath. Then my chest opened up, my lungs opened up, and I could smell things again.

I had ten sessions, one a week, and I tell people those were the best ten weeks of my life. Not just looking back but during those sessions, I knew the changes were wonderful and wondered why I had waited so long.

I had always had a very low tolerance to pain. My first ten sessions were powerful, and there was pain involved with each one. I never enjoyed it, but I began to understand that pain isn't so bad and was no longer afraid of it. That was a wonderful and powerful realization. I remember at first that I would close my eyes and go into an altered state. I didn't like that. It wasn't comfortable. I don't even think that is what Rolfing is all about. I believe it is about being here, now and aware. When I kept my eyes open I could see how patterns and my vision changed.

During the sessions in Colorado, we would focus on a particular group of muscles and go right at them. I would learn different options of movement with each muscle. I would move one knee clockwise or counterclockwise while keeping the other knee still. I could feel the difference. We also worked on the whole body. If you tell a Rolfer you have a problem with your knee, they will start working on your ear because it's all connected.

I will probably continue to get Rolfed when I have problems or when I am trying to get to a different point in my riding. I use it as a tool to help me with the horses and am sure it helps in other parts of my life too. I am relaxed after a session and ready to get organized. The Rolfer helps organize my body, but I in turn try to organize my finances, my social activities and achieve a balance in my life.

Every time I get Rolfing sessions I see, smell and hear better. I can come in with an allergy and have the sniffles and go out without the feeling of fluid in my face. Everything opens up. Also, I can tolerate the hay, straw, and mold from the dust better afterward.

After I had the first ten Rolfing sessions, it was wild how I saw a tree in my own yard I never knew was there. I noticed the fields are plowed in rectangles. Realizations popped into my brain. I don't think I ever looked at the sky before. Maybe I saw a star or two, but I never noticed the different patterns in the sky or was aware of the different levels of brightness of the sun throughout the day. I am much more aware of my environment now.

Petey's Turn

I've been working with horses since the age of ten. I breed, train, buy and sell them and am also a professional riding instructor. Rolfing was such a positive experience for me that I wanted to see if it would unlock some structural problems in Petey, a four-year-old mare that I raised. Petey was stiff and tense. She was nervous of strangers, new things and generally fearful of the world. Sometimes when she was ridden she went under the saddle, causing a splint or formation of calcium on the cannon bones in her front legs. She jarred her legs too hard.

I asked Briah to work on Petey. At first Petey was suspicious of what we were doing, but as Briah worked on her head, Petey's eyelids got heavier and she appeared to be tranquilized. Their rapport began immediately after that. It was a bonding experience for both of them.

As Briah worked on Petey's poll, the top part of a horse's neck down to the lower part of the neck, I had my hands on the mare and could feel the Rolfing going through her body. We took a picture of her then, and her head, which had been high in the air from being startled, was down below my kneecaps. She had relaxed so much that her head went way down to the ground. This is the way a horse shows trust.

When Briah started working at the top of Petey's shoulder, she needed more leverage, so Briah got on top of Petey and worked downward on the muscles. As Briah worked on the side of Petey's neck, the veins became more prominent. I could actually see the blood circulating and her breathing becoming deeper. The barn animals all came over to watch when Briah started working. She worked for two hours on Petey, climbing all over her and at one point using a ladder to get leverage. It was intense work, and Briah would have to rest for hours afterward.

After five sessions, Petey's coat became lighter and healthier. It remained lighter for the rest of the time that I owned her. In the "after" pictures that we took of her, she has a longer neck, and her muscles are more pronounced. She's standing more upright on her legs instead of her legs being sort of sprawled out like a baby horse would stand. She had big, thick muscles on the under part of her neck from tensing up so often, and they are beginning to go away. Her neck is no longer underslung. She has some pretty muscles coming out on top of her neck now. She's more alert after five sessions in terms of using her ears and eyes, her collar, and the way she's standing up.

Before Rolfing, Petey looked like a barnyard horse. Now she's bright and alert like a show horse. She stands base wide, centered perfectly over the tops of her feet. Her legs come straight down rather than spreading out. In the before pictures, she is standing on the outside of her feet, like some people walk, and in the after pictures, you can tell that she's standing right over the center, on the tops of her feet. Her weight is shifted back to her hocks, making her look more capable of bearing weight and producing more athletic movements. Her rhythm at trotting is synchronized now, and because her shoulders are freed up, she uses

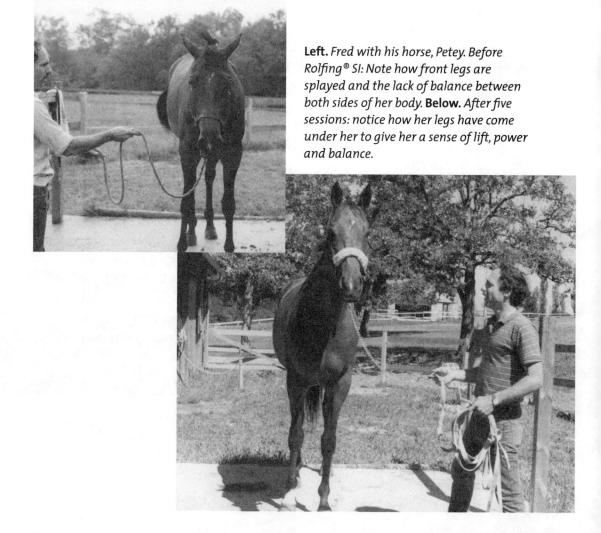

Left. *Fred with his horse, Petey. Before Rolfing® SI: Note how front legs are splayed and the lack of balance between both sides of her body.* **Below.** *After five sessions: notice how her legs have come under her to give her a sense of lift, power and balance.*

them more effectively. Less restriction in her hind quarters has significantly improved her jumping.

Observations

Petey seemed to love the Rolfing sessions and afterward would be relaxed and appear to vibrate positive energy. As she opened up in the chest, I could tell that a lot of intense energy was being released. It was very powerful.

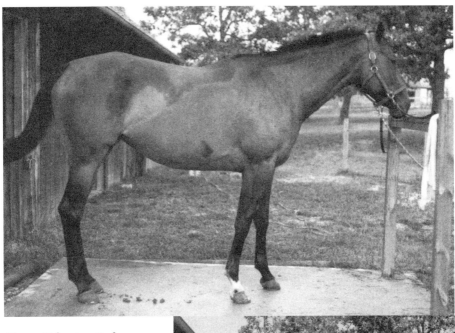

Above. *Side view. Before Rolfing® SI: Note the lack of alignment and support from both her front and rear legs. Note how each segment of her body seems compressed and disconnected.* **Right.** *After five Sessions: note how Petey has lengthened through her body and looks collected and integrated. Her legs are squarely under her and she looks solid, balanced, and younger.*

Now when I ride Petey she puts her head down for the bridle and stands quietly while I tighten the girth on the saddle. Her overall attitude is more amiable. She is more likable and likes everything a lot more.

House's Turn

Briah also worked on another horse, one named House because he is so wonderfully big. He's really come a long way. She worked on House twice for several hours each time. He loves people and was very trusting. House had a terribly short neck that was inhibiting his jumping style and movement. He did learn to stretch out and stretch down into the bit. Before, he was so far behind the bit that it threw his balance off. The Rolfing facilitated the training. Now he seems so huge; I have to stretch my elbows out, he's so long.

The Rolfing process holds a lot of potential for horses. There are a lot of body adjustments and chiropractics with horses at the racetrack, and riders have always used various kinds of body work because riding is so hard on the body. The Rolfing process, though, hasn't yet caught on. I don't know many Rolfers that work with horses, but the benefits are great. The horse has less risk of injury because its body is aligned and more relaxed, but if an injury does occur, the recuperation is quicker. Rolfing also improves the horse's performance, and I know from my own experience that it also improves that of the rider.

I would really like to see Rolfing workshops set up with the local equestrian teams. Whether the horse gets the work or the rider gets it, it seems to help everything else. It builds self-confidence and creates a sense of well-being that is essential for a good performance. I'm interested in the self-confidence that Rolfing provides, especially with horses because when the horse feels a sense of well-being, I think they perform at higher levels. I saw that in the two horses that Briah worked on.

House: wonderfully big. A gorgeous example of Rolfing® SI success!

The Professional Athlete:
Maintaining High Performance

Lisa Daley, on her dog Phoenix

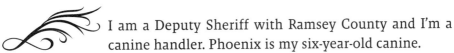 I am a Deputy Sheriff with Ramsey County and I'm a canine handler. Phoenix is my six-year-old canine.

As a canine police dog, Phoenix, like me, is expected to perform at the drop of a hat. We could be six hours into our shift and he could be lying in the back of the kennel sleeping, and then in a split second, he has to act fast and act physically. He has to keep going for as long as we are tracking suspects. He has to be able to track while dealing with obstacles and even ice. He needs to be able to have the endurance to last and to find the bad guy, and then to do it all over again, and sometimes even do it yet again if need be. We have eight-hour shifts, but there have been times when I have had to call upon him in the heat to do several calls— for tracking, a building search, or to do a drug search. Anything that he is asked to do (and being a dog who loves to work), he will do it. As soon as I say go, he will do it even if he is not feeling well.

I heard about Rolfing® through Beth Miller, the neuromuscular masseuse who works on me. I told her that I was having some problems with my canine, Phoenix, and she recommended Briah.

Phoenix had been limping. At the time I did not know it, but he had elbow dysplasia. After I had him Rolfed I took him to a chiropractor for an adjustment. He still had a little of the limp, so I took him in to the University of Minnesota veterinarians where they found that he has some dysplasia in his elbow.

Now mind you, Phoenix is not just your average dog. He is a hundred-pound black German shepherd and very athletic. He is not overweight. Technically, he is a professional athlete. That being said, I noticed that after the Rolfing he was less sluggish. Now the average person looking at him would not be able to tell that he was less sluggish. But he is a canine police dog and I train and work with him all the time, so I noticed this minor sluggishness and that he wasn't as peppy. It looked to me like he just didn't feel 100 percent. Dogs can't talk so you have to learn to read them, and what I was reading was that it was his front right elbow that was giving him this sluggishness. I think that an injury affects your whole body, and that dealing with this elbow problem had led to his lack of pep. After he was Rolfed, it looked like all of his problems were gone except for his elbow and that's all he had to deal with. He looked good. He had the spring back in his step and he was ready to work again.

It seems that with Phoenix no one therapy by itself was able to bring him back 100 percent; to make it 100 percent he needed the Rolfing work, the chiropractic work and the vet work. With this combination of therapies I feel that I can give him a full, healthy, long-lasting life. I am hoping he will feel good for the rest of his life, and I will get a good ten years of work from him with this kind of care.

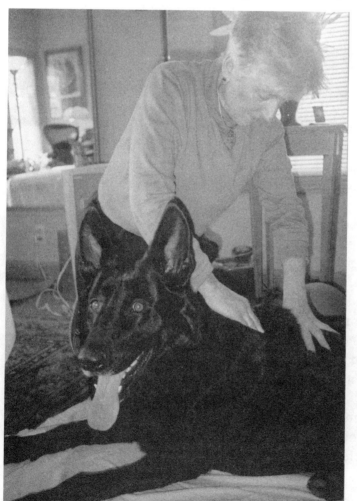

Phoenix, a six-year-old German shepherd, enjoying the benefits of Rolfing® SI. Releasing stress and imbalance maintains his high performance as a Canine Police Dog.

Phoenix's Rolfing SI Sessions

Phoenix had three Rolfing sessions last year. After the first I could see the difference. We do a lot of training and preparation for the summer work, and being an athlete myself I know that not just one session is good enough. He needed to get the first session in and I needed to see how he did with that. He did wonderfully with it, so I got another session for him to make sure it took and to get him ready for the summer.

In the summer, we put a lot of pressure on our canines and a lot of work, because we have to do our annual certification to make them eligible for street work. This entails one regional trial which is generally around the end of June, and then the national trials which are in September. In 2007, our team took first in the country, and then in 2008 we took second, so we are going back this year to get that trophy back.

In the regional trials you have to get a minimum score to certify in order to have your dog eligible to work the street. Its governing agency is called the USPCA—the United States Police Canine Association. Within this association are actual handlers who work the street, and it is these same handlers that judge you and the dogs.

These regional trials include events for obedience and agility. Agility events include: four or five hurdles to jump, an eight-foot wall to scale, a ladder to climb, and a cat walk which can be especially hard on an ageing dog's body. These events require great balance, agility, strength, and discipline. Then there are the apprehension events which are fun and games for them. These include a suspect search, which consists of six boxes with a person hiding in one of them. They have to find the suspect which is the easy part. The hard part is that there is also what we call a hot box, which is where the suspect was on the last hide. Now the dog has to differentiate between the fresh scent and the hot scent—and they do. They hit on both scents and they know that there is scent here, but this scent over there is different, and that is where the person is.

In September at the nationals, Phoenix was phenomenal. I'm kind of biased, but he really was phenomenal. In 2008 we were sixteenth out of 120 dogs so we made the top twenty. If you make the top twenty in the country you're considered to be in the top. You're top dog, very top dog.

The difference between his performance a year ago, before all this fresh input of the Rolfing, and his performance this year, can be compared to the difference between a professional marathon runner and someone who's just beginning to run. That is the difference in terms of his level of ability and performance. It's not just a physical balance that Rolfing did for him, it's an all-around balancing.

Mentally, he's even more alert. There is a smoothness to him. It has enabled his full strength, full body, and full mind to be used. If he hadn't had the Rolfing I don't think his full potential would have ever come out, or it would have already. At this age his full potential would have been past and he would be on the downhill slide. Whereas now, even at six years of age, I think he still has better years ahead.

Phoenix has always been a pretty remarkable dog. Whenever people look at him, they comment. But in the last few years since I've been getting Rolfing sessions for him, I get even more comments along this line. In fact, one of the head vets at the University commented that he is the fittest dog she has ever seen—*ever*. Those are her words, I'm not exaggerating. She didn't explain, but I believe she meant that in looking at Phoenix, he just looks fit—very put together and strong. We were just looking at him trying to figure out why he had this very slight limp. She didn't even feel him, but even with this limp she said that this was the fittest dog she had ever seen.

He is just healthy all around. I believe it is partly a result of what I do with him, but the Rolfing has definitely played a big part.

There are ten police dogs in our department. Compared to those other dogs, I think Phoenix feels better. There are three I could pick out that need Rolfing! They could use an adjustment as well. They need work, and I can tell that by their walk. I see imbalances translating into the dogs feeling uncomfortable, so they're not as sharp or at ease as they could be. Getting Rolfing for Phoenix has helped me see these kinds of differences, and I can tell it is the time of year that Phoenix is due for a visit to Briah. I have had him adjusted but again, that's not the complete package. He needs some Rolfing sessions to bring everything together and bring out that potential. Once he's had a session I know I'll see a difference immediately. He becomes energized in a very positive way and that tells me he is feeling good.

The Working Dog

The Rolfing work helps Phoenix concentrate and do his work efficiently. Yesterday is a good example. We were invited along when the gang strike force did a search warrant at an address in Vadnais Heights. Phoenix gets pretty wild and worked up, thinking it's man work, that he's going to get a bite or an apprehension, or he's going to find a bad guy. I initially thought that's what we were there for too. We sat in the back yard when they went in on the search warrant, and if anyone ran out the back door Phoenix would apprehend him. But everything was secure so we had to put that aside. We were called inside and Phoenix had to do his drug search. To start with, he was still in apprehension mode and not searching for drugs, and I had to change his mindset. I had to put him in a sit, calm him down, and then tell him seek dope. This helps him make the switch and figure out we are doing something different now. If a

dog is not feeling well or they are in pain or they haven't been Rolfed, it takes a lot more effort to make that switch. The handler may have to take the dog outside, put him in the car for a little bit, and let him calm down, before trying the drug search. But Phoenix can switch now without all that effort. This is part of the Rolfing process, too. As we integrate the neuromuscular system he is more able to switch quickly. It's all a part of his whole being.

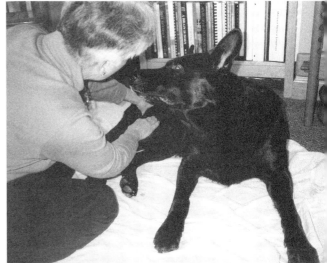

I also pay a lot of attention to making sure that his nutrition is really good, and that's also very important for tissue health and mental well-being. Exercise is also necessary, just as it is for humans. Some of the officers don't work their dogs physically as much as I do, especially the older they get. With Phoenix, the older he gets the more I do to take care of him and exercise him well.

"Once he's had a session, I know I'll see a difference immediately. He becomes energized in a very positive way and that tells me he is feeling good."

RAMSEY COUNTY DEPUTY SHERIFF, LISA DALEY

For people who have working dogs or agility dogs, Rolfing is invaluable. Phoenix is my partner but he's also my pet, and I take him home where I have other personal pets. If you want to get the most out of your relationship with your pet, you need to take care of them. It's just like my husband: if I want to get the most out of my relationship with him, I want him to take care of himself, feel good, and get the things done that need doing. With my pets, I have to initiate that. If you want the best out of their short little lives, then you need to do what needs to be done.

The typical lifespan for a German Shepherd is eleven to twelve years, thirteen at the most. Those last few years may not be high quality, but if I keep taking care of Phoenix he'll feel good longer, and if I listen to what he's trying to tell me, I will be able to know when he needs more Rolfing and adjustments. Hopefully, he'll live longer than normal with a good quality of life. That's what it's all about—I want him to have the best quality of life possible for him. The Rolfing is a big piece of that puzzle along with the chiropractic work, good food, exercise, and good vet care.

Rebuilding the Awkward Horse

Briah relates her work with Prelude at Walnut Hill Farm,
Greenwood, Missouri, 1996

Prelude was an eight-year-old Trakehner (a German gelding) that was ridden as a hunter jumper and was now
learning dressage. His owner, Jan Smith, had bought him as a hunter a
couple of years before and said that he had competed very successfully in
the hunter ring.

When both Jan and Jennifer (her daughter, an accomplished rider)
rode Prelude, they could feel his resistance to accepting the bit and he
would not come through on his right rear side. This made it difficult
for him to support the rider with his back consistently or stay supple,
forward, and bent going in either direction (to the left or right). Prelude
would not move forward or maintain an open and free base because he
was not able to do it comfortably. He became a sluggish, lethargic horse
at a walk, trot, canter, and unwilling to give more impulsion. Since he
was not able to remain consistent and rhythmic, the rider would always
have to adapt to a less than energetic and inconsistent gait.

Prelude would tire easily and the training process broke down his
body rather than the training enhancing his body and movement. It
made his back sore, and he was unwilling to give because of pain. He
became stiff and short in the twenty minutes of warm-up prior to training actually starting.

Why Rolfing® Structural Integration?

My previous experience of doing Rolfing® Structural Integration with a
number of horses showed me that Rolfing SI can shorten the warm-up
time, and enable the horse to move more freely and move forward much

more willingly and immediately. I felt that Prelude's gait would become cleaner, more clearly articulated, and that each leg would move independently and straight-track correctly. I also felt that he would be able to engage his legs, hind end, offer more of his back, and be able to stretch his neck and top line forward.

Jan had been through the Rolfing SI process and knew that she felt better, freer and more balanced. She felt that Prelude wasn't moving up to his potential so she decided to get some Rolfing SI sessions for him. She felt that this could be a wonderful experience for both horse and rider. Since he was a young and athletic horse, he had a lot of potential but he certainly was not using his body up to his potential.

I decided to mentor Jan's daughter, Jennifer, and have her assist me with the sessions. Jennifer is an accomplished and beautiful rider and had been through the Rolfing SI process so she had a good level of organization and integration in her own structure. She is also a Certified Rolfer™ and has a deep understanding of the application of this work to horses. The following are notes from our collaboration together.

Session One

Analysis of Movement
On the lunge line, the first time he was going to the left, his left front leg was moving shorter than the right front leg. The left rear leg looked especially short and contracted, particularly in the stifle area. This leg tended to cross the midline and his rear legs were not under his pelvis. This means that because of this structural problem, he couldn't get his legs to propel and support his back. Without support from his hind end, his front end had to pull the hind end along. This caused additional tightness and contraction in the shoulder girdle. Because of this pattern, the neck and head also pulled short into the shoulder girdle. The gait that resulted from this structural pattern was short and stiff.

The Session
The first goal was to open up Prelude's breathing. The chest area was worked with particular attention to freeing the neck from the chest, the withers, and the shoulder girdle with some work down into the front legs. We did some superficial work along the spine. The next area of emphasis was working the area where the hip joint joins into the pelvis. The goal was to free the rear legs from the pelvis, thereby creating more

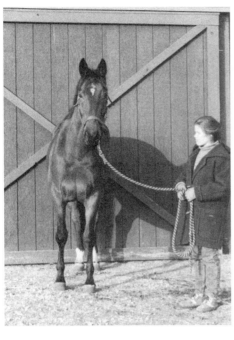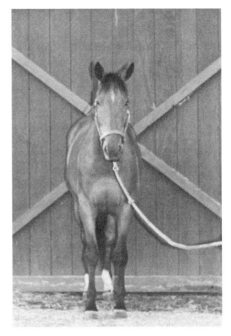

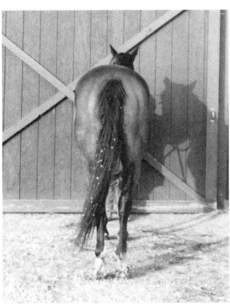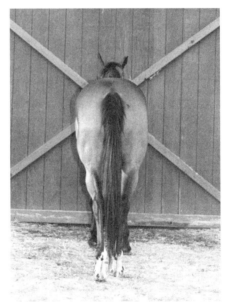

Top left. *Before Rolfing® SI (with Jennifer Smith) Prelude, not squarely aligned in his structure.* **Top right.** *After five Sessions: shows his head and neck nicely aligned with the rest of his structure.*

Bottom left. *Rear View: Before session one: Note the imbalance in his hind end. The left side is higher, there is a lack of balance and symmetry and the overdeveloped musculature that is compressed and thick.* **Bottom right.** *After five sessions: you can now draw a vertical line from the middle of the tail through the center of his head. His legs are more integrated into his pelvis and there is now a sense of balance and symmetry.*

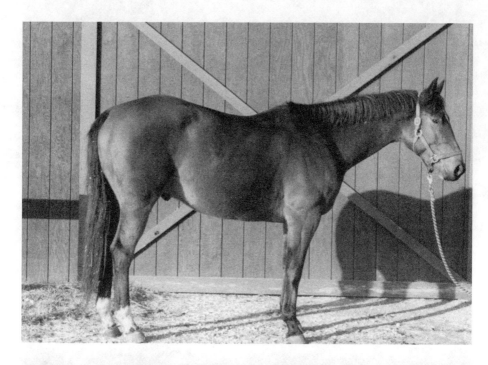

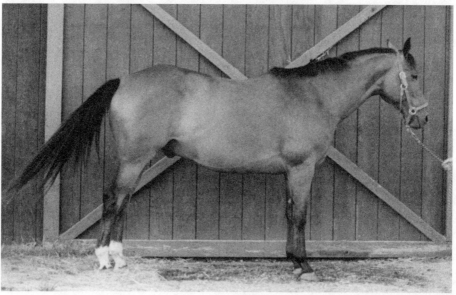

Top. *Before Session one: A look of tightness and compression.* **Bottom.** *After five sessions: Prelude is bigger, fuller, more squarely aligned with a much younger and athletic look to him.*

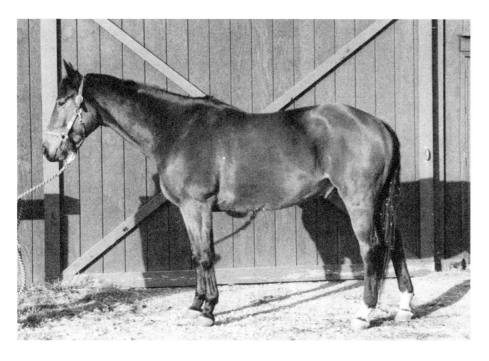

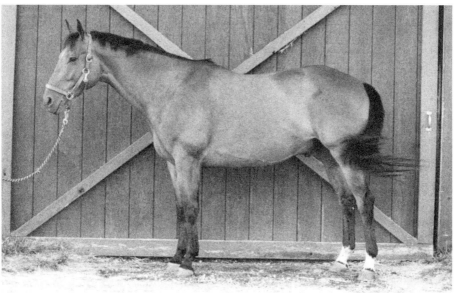

Top. *Before session one: Compression and tightness again.* **Bottom.** *After five sessions: Note the fuller body and natural alignment.*

space for the legs to move back more freely from the pelvis. A little more work was done in the pelvic floor as a way to provide more space and separation of the legs from the pelvis.

Observations

As we started the work on his chest, he stretched his neck and lifted his head up and out, leading his movement with his muzzle, giving a real sense of lifting outward from the chest. As we worked the shoulder, he would move and shift his weight as he balanced the motion we created in his musculature. It was most interesting to observe that as we worked the area of the shoulders, for example, he would constantly be shifting all four legs in a very conscious and particular way, providing an extension of the work that was being done up above into far regions below in his feet. What came alive was seeing how mobile Prelude was, and what a natural rhythm emerged from within him as we worked with him. Often he assisted us by leaning into us so that not only could we work deeper, but he would also actively integrate the work by extending out of the pattern and back into balance. This was the dynamic flow of the session: there was a constant interaction and flow between our movements and his movements, always resulting in all four legs shifting to a better position under his body.

Jennifer was struck by the innate quality of movement in the tissue where we could see that a little stimulation from us created waves of change all through his structure. A little went a long way!

Early on in the Rolfing SI process, there was a definite relaxation, yet a real alertness in his attention and tracking with everything we were doing. Even when we pulled up a chair on one side and a heavy bench on the other, this didn't seem to faze him. His whole demeanor was cooperative, inviting the work, and generally looking "blissed out." His eyes were glazed over. He looked as though he had just been awakened from a heavy nap and acted a little groggy. The next morning when Jennifer went to feed him, he was parched and drank a lot of water. This is typical with people after Rolfing SI. In creating more layers of freed up tissues, the tissues are literally thirsty for hydration. Day one and the day after this session, he seemed more interested in his grain. Prior to Rolfing SI, Prelude's pattern around food was to eat all his hay and to not finish all his grain. At this point he had a bigger appetite.

Before this session, Jennifer had noticed that there was a lot of undigested grain in his manure. Another observation she made is that when she rode Prelude he would lift his tail and act as if he needed to defecate. She felt it as a sudden syncopation in gait. This is not an unusual pattern with Prelude. It is as if he had to defecate and couldn't. It may have indicated some amount of constipation or, with a rider is on his back, it created enough pressure that he was unable to naturally release and defecate. After being cooled down and while waiting to be turned out, he always passed manure. This happened almost every time Prelude was ridden.

Session Two, Two Weeks Later

Before the Session
We put Prelude on the lunge line so we could observe his movement patterns since the last session. Prelude seemed more alert, present and willing to go forward. There was more extension in the shoulders and front legs as well as more fluid movement of his neck and head extending forward through space. What became apparent was that his hindquarters looked caught up from the pelvic girdle to the croup. It was as if there was a tight band around his pelvic girdle that was restricting his movement. We noticed that his hind legs were not crossing the midline as much as before the first session. He looked as if he might want to buck, but lacked the overall coordination or will to try in the small circle.

The Session
Based on what we observed of Prelude on the lunge line, we focused our attention and work first on freeing the band around his pelvic girdle. We worked the croup (basically all the rotators, etc), did some work around the pelvic floor and inside the groin area. We worked the body of the neck and then focused our work on freeing the relationship of the neck to the head. We then did some integration and worked the area just on either side of the spine all the way back to the tail. This summarizes the general areas that were addressed in this session.

After the Session
Prelude was put back on the lunge line and photographs were taken to record his process in movement. When first put on the lunge line, Prelude was sort of timid and wasn't quite sure where his feet belonged. He was still in an altered state from two hours of Rolfing SI. He still wasn't moving forward, so in order to encourage him Jennifer asked him to

canter. The effect she wanted was for Prelude to go forward openly at a quicker gait and then asked him to go into a downward transition back to the trot without taking away the energy of the canter. I had the sense that he was beginning to feel the Rolfing SI integrate, and he integrated it into a more articulated movement in his hindquarters.

This was immediately followed by an increased ability in his hind legs to track up in line with his front legs, and move into a more extended trot. As he continued to become more accustomed to the feeling of his new balance, he became more confident in moving forward. He did not look stiff and strained in his shoulders, rather he willingly reached forward and enjoyed the floating suspension in the trot. He looked like he was surprising himself in his newfound ability to move freely. He even bucked and raced around. The increased energy and relaxation from the session made him feel more agile and the bucking was no problem.

Jennifer had the sense that before the session, he would have lost his balance had he tried to buck, and possibly fallen. Jan observed that all his musculature was rippling in his hindquarters, and he seemed stiff and sore. He almost always expected the rider to slam on his back. This was changing as he became more comfortable with offering his back, and the rider could sit on him more comfortably.

The Week Following the Rolfing SI Session
Jennifer rode Prelude three times, the first day without supervision. She felt slightly different movement in him during the first ride. His willingness to go forward was apparent but without the trainer's eye and cues, she felt she was not accessing the potential of his movement. There is always the problem of a rider not being able to "see" what is really happening with a horse from the ground. The trainer's function is to see and pull the picture together.

The next day she was able to ride in a structured lesson. The trainer started making Jennifer more aware of where she and the horse were in relationship to one another. Then Jennifer could develop the awareness and the "feel" of when she and Prelude were in harmony, or when they were not. The focus of the lesson was on building the trot. Before, when Prelude would circle to the left he would slant, fall to the inside, and not use his right hind leg. As a result, Jennifer would fall to the left, collapsing, making the left sitz bone ineffectual and compounding the problem. The trainer cued Jennifer to straighten herself upright, take the feel of the outside, right rein, tap his hind (right leg) with the whip and demand that he engage it. For the first time, Prelude really squared himself up, took his weight on the outside right leg and pushed off forward in balance. This immediately gave the pair a new sensation and actualized their movement into a more harmonious uplifting trot. The potential for forwardness, straightness, and the feeling of Prelude offering his back and hindquarters was becoming a reality.

The next day, the pair worked with less supervision but started to warm up with a feeling that they were taking off from where they ended in the lesson the day before. Jennifer still needed to adjust herself and remembered to stay supple and keep her hip angle open and flexible. Prelude moved more confidently forward, more comfortable and assured that he was not going to feel pain if he moved forward. He seemed to make the realizations of the day before seem like his normal way of moving. The ride felt more effortless. Prelude was balanced, and supple in his body, neck and head. Every step was more courageous and confident than the last. This resulted in Prelude filling up the bridle "in harmony" with Jennifer's request to move forward and laterally in leg-yields with subtle cues. He was happier and more compliant to work since he was no longer in pain.

The final assessment of this ride was that Prelude was in tune with Jennifer and vice versa. The two seemed to be able to stay in harmony while executing movements (like leg-yields) which before were inconsistent, choppy and lacking forwardness. The feeling of confidence and trust between the pair became part of their new working relationship. Before, it seemed as if Prelude was expecting an inconsistent "bad" ride; now their moments of harmony and being in tune brought them both the confidence to work together. The pair exhibited a picture of dancing together, Jennifer leading and Prelude following with more confidence.

Session Three, a Week Later

The Session
We chose to work with Prelude in his stall in the main barn as it was a warmer environment. The temperature was less than 30 degrees. There were several riders preparing their horses and riding in the adjacent indoor arena; and consequently, it took Prelude quite a while to settle down and get centered.

One of Prelude's weaknesses is his tendency to become easily distracted due to his own nervousness and anxiety. This tendency impacts his ability to respond appropriately to the call for engagement. This also affects his ability to relax fully through the movements that are necessary for dressage.

In retrospect, working in his stall with all the distractions may have enabled him to reframe his anxiety. It took about forty-five minutes to get him into an altered state where he began to restructure his reaction to the multidimensional stimuli (horses, riders, trainers, interruptions). Hopefully, he will be able to take this experience into the ring when he is being ridden.

Rolfing SI restructures the newer muscular patterns and allows the person/animal to access a deeper state of relaxation which eliminates random movements and reactions to stimuli. The fight or flight syndrome present in all animals, is reduced from a reactionary response to a more sensible, trainable pattern of behavior. Rolfing SI facilitates a deeper level of human/animal bonding and mutual trust. It also normalizes random reactionary behavior to a more organized and predictable integration of behavior and movement.

More in-depth work was done to balance and square the shoulder girdle. Particular attention was spent on bringing more symmetry into the neck-to-chest relationship. The result of this in-depth work was that we were able to get his head and neck squarely aligned onto his shoulder girdle. The other area of emphasis was in squaring off the pelvic girdle. Particular attention was focused on the inner line of his rear legs (the adductor and hamstring compartments) and freeing the legs from the pelvis. The above work took two practitioners about three hours of intense and consistent work.

After the Session

We asked Aaron, the trainer, to ride Prelude immediately after the session. By having a professional trainer that has a solid position and clearly focused intentions for the ride, we felt we would be able to observe Prelude's integration of the work under more exacting conditions. This gave us the opportunity to sit back and watch as Prelude came close to reaching his movement potential.

Observations

We observed an increased willingness to go forward. Aaron stated that he did not have to push Prelude forward. The energy level of the ride was consistent and of an adequate pace, whereas before, his tempo was somewhat inconsistent and a little sluggish. We also observed more articulation and movement in the hocks.

All joint movements were functioning so well that the impact of his movement through space was a picture of a horse moving in slow motion. There was a sense of harmony and well-equilibrated motion that was smooth and rhythmical. It was very inspiring to watch!

Four days later, Jennifer rode Prelude and found that he engaged effortlessly and continued to offer more, physically and mentally, during the ride. For example, he never resisted her commands or fell apart as he would have previous to the Rolfing SI process. We discovered that now we did not know what Prelude's true potential might actually be. His structure and function were now so different that we felt that we now had a new horse that might go farther than previously thought with his training.

Session Four, Two Weeks Later

The Session

The focus of this session was to release the legs from the pelvis and to integrate the hind legs into the pelvis and back. We worked the circle around the flank on both sides; the medial attachments of the adductors to the pelvis; the pelvic floor; and spent quite some time organizing and freeing the hamstrings. To finish the session, we did some integrating work to lengthen the muscles along the spine on both sides. This was slow, tedious work in an area that was thick and compact. There are so many layers of musculature in the pelvis of a horse and since it is the main engine for movement, there was a tremendous amount of "beefy" work to be executed.

Observations

Prelude is increasingly making himself more available to change and to receiving the work. At the beginning of the first sessions, he would sometimes be unfocused and difficult to engage until halfway through the session, then finally succumb to a deeper state of relaxation. With this fourth session, we led him out of the stall, tied him to a hitching post and each began working. Within moments he was immediately in a trance or hypnotic state; still conscious but allowing his eyelids to become droopy, his eyes became glazed over, his lips open and quivering, and his breathing became very deep and rhythmical with sighs and release. He moved his body as we worked on him, illustrating the horse's ability to use their inner intelligence to absorb and integrate the work immediately.

He seemed to work with us better away from other horses, when he had our full attention and less distraction from other horses. After the session we decided to put him in a paddock and free lunge him. He bucked and exploded into a gallop as if he was letting off an abundance of energy. Jan commented that this was unusual for Prelude as he is not an excitable horse and usually just trotted off to eat grass.

Session Five, Three Weeks Later

The Session
For this last session we did some opening in his pelvic girdle, and worked again to get more opening in his shoulder girdle so he could have more space for movement through his whole body. Once this was accomplished, I focused on integrating his head to neck connection; neck to shoulder system, giving him more length along either side of his spine and body; then some final integration through all four legs.

Again, with Jennifer and I working together, we were able to bring about some beautiful changes. This session was efficiently performed and Prelude seemed to know exactly what his role in this cooperative venture was.

Observations
After the session we lined Prelude up in the same location and stance that we had photographed him in the before-Rolfing SI photos. In the before photos he is not squarely lined up with himself. The after-five photo shows his head and neck nicely aligned with the rest of his structure. There is a sense of balance and symmetry which the before photograph does not show. The photos of the rear side also reveal the imbalance that was traveling through his structure. The left side of his pelvis is higher and his musculature is bound up. In the post-sessions photo, both sides of his body are much more balanced, aligned and symmetrical. There is a vertical line that is now visible from the center of his head, through his body and out his tail.

The side-view photos reveal the results of the work. In the right profile before photo, Prelude does not look very well put together. There is a general look of tightness and compression going through all his major segments (head to neck to shoulder, through his body and into his hind end). The after-five photos of both of his sides show a horse that has lengthened through each segment. He is bigger, fuller, and all the lines extend throughout his neck, head, and through to his pelvis. His legs are more squarely aligned under him and his pelvis has much more integrity and balance. He now has a well aligned structure with a much younger and athletic look to him.

Last Thoughts

A local television crew came out to do a story on Prelude and the Rolfing SI process and Jan was asked to sum up her observations on the results of the Rolfing SI. She commented that after the Rolfing SI Prelude came into his own. He all of a sudden was balanced, he began to move more freely and seemed to use the back end that he needs to power the engine. She has been getting wonderful compliments on how he looks and how effortlessly he moves. She stated that he won the championship in his first dressage show a month ago after his Rolfing SI in Kansas City. She said, "I see a much happier relaxed attitude in the horse. He's not in pain. He feels good, and after Briah finished working on him, (he's not a terribly energetic horse, he doesn't want to go out and throw himself around because it takes too much work) Prelude will now go out and be frisky like a two-year-old, like our baby colt. He will go out and throw himself around like he feels so good."

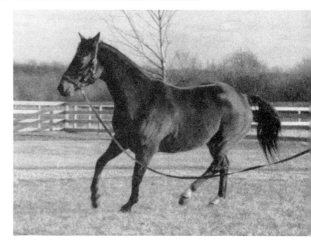

Before Rolfing® SI: On the lunge line—demonstrating his compression and difficulty with moving forward.

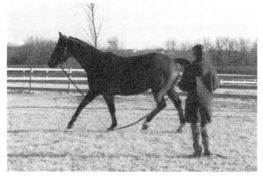

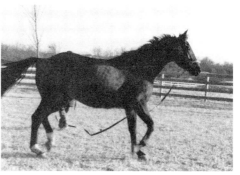

As a demonstration for the news story, I did a few minutes of Rolfing SI with Prelude, and then Jennifer rode him to illustrate how he now moves. The TV commentator asked what I observed after these five sessions, and if I saw success. I replied, "Absolutely. It's the difference between seeing a horse that moved like a little sewing machine—hard on his feet—and now he is very, very light. Now he looks like he is barely touching down. It is really beautiful. This is a finale to an incredible process with this horse. He looks like he is several sizes larger and fuller; there is beautiful extension in all his lines. He moves through space like a beautiful athlete and dancer."

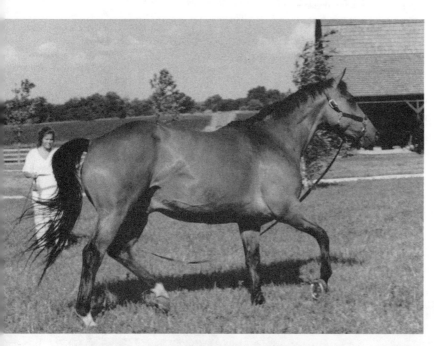

After five sessions: Coming into his own. He is now balanced and able to move freely and powerfully like a beautiful athlete-dancer.

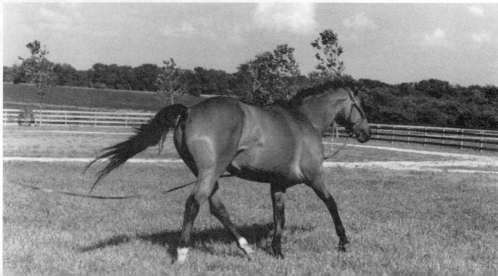

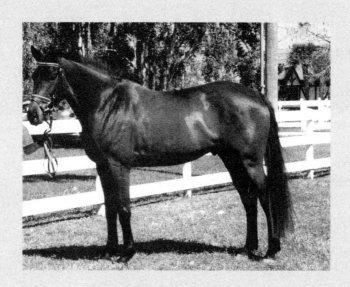

Cappuccino

Cappuccino, a three-year old Holsteiner
gelding, received Rolfing® SI just hours after
birth, and three sessions within two months.
"Cappy" is elegant, balanced, and has three
excellent gaits. He is shown here as a sport
horse/dressage prospect.

Photo courtesy of Jan Smith

Maintaining the Athletic Edge

Kim Makie, on her Airedale, Toni

I had a number of Rolfing® sessions myself, and it helped me in a number of ways. Initially I had come because I had always felt that my body had a twist in it which showed up as one shoulder lower than the other. I attributed this to all the different sports I had played through high school and college: basketball, tennis, volleyball, softball, golf, weightlifting, and biking. I had put my body through a lot of different stresses, but luckily I had no major injuries to speak of. I did have a sense of being compact, though—tenser, tighter than I wanted to be.

After the Rolfing series I was looser, less compact and more flexible. After just the first session my shoulders became level. I had lived with that unevenness for years, thinking that was just how I was. I didn't have that sense of twisting that I had had. I had fewer injuries, too, which is important to me as I get older as it seems to take a little longer to heal now. I just feel more physically sound. For at a period of time after I've had a few Rolfing sessions, I feel straighter when I walk, and people tell me that I walk more upright. I've lost my stoop. Rolfing has become something that I do periodically because I've become more attuned to feeling when I start to revert back. When I start to feel that tension and torque in my body, I know that I need to get it straightened out before it causes problems.

I got my Airedale, Toni, when she was four years old from a breeder who had tried unsuccessfully to breed her. She had lived with three or four other dogs in a house, and during the day they had been kept in crates. They were let out in the evening but for a large part of the time they were cooped up in crates.

When I got Toni, I noticed that she didn't like to sit down. It seemed really uncomfortable for her to sit and it became even more noticeable when I took her to dog training. I would try to get her to do a sit, but I could tell that something was hurting. It wasn't that she didn't want to do it, but it was uncomfortable. It looked like one of her legs was too tight, which might have been caused by being corked up in that crate and not running around. I thought that by exercising her more she would get more comfortable, but after about a year I noticed she still did not like to sit.

I took her to my vet but he couldn't find anything wrong structurally or skeletally that might have caused the problem. Luckily for Toni, he is pretty conservative. Some veterinarians might have put her on an anti-inflammatory or given her cortisone, but this veterinarian doesn't work that way. I'm active enough with her that I just didn't want her to have the pain, so I thought I would try something else.

Because of the loosening and flexibility I'd gained from the Rolfing process, I thought maybe it could have the same effect on Toni. I brought her in to Briah and she seemed to take to the session pretty well. She is not a really hyper dog, but she quickly became pretty comfortable and relaxed. Briah worked on Toni's hip, which she could tell was tighter, and then she had me feel it. As Briah moved it a certain way, I could feel the hip get even tighter.

Briah gave her three sessions, and that was five years ago. To this day she has had no problems sitting. She can sit and lie down easily so whatever was causing the problem is just not there any more.

Before the pain disappeared she had a kind of tight personality—probably from dealing with the pain. Now she is a more relaxed and mellow dog. Airedales are known for being tightly wound with a hyper nervous system, but Toni was always calm for an Airedale to begin with. Even so, there is a very noticeable difference in how relaxed she is now that she isn't in pain. That was the big thing, and that has remained. Those three sessions balanced her out emotionally, not just physically. It's not that she can't get excited if she sees something, but overall she's extremely calm.

Briah had shown me how I could work on her at home, so off and on I would work that area for her. To this day, when I touch that area she just relaxes, and she'll let me gently rub the area and move her leg. Before the Rolfing sessions she would not have allowed that, and somehow this work has helped her understand that this is good for her. I think she's just more attuned to touch than she was before. She didn't necessarily like touch before, and I'm guessing that it hurt. Now she's really an affectionate dog. She will cuddle right up next to me and she loves to be massaged, which is something I couldn't do to her when I first got her.

Airedales only live to about twelve. Toni is nine years old now and very active—she's more like a five- or six-year-old dog. She doesn't seem to have any pain, nor is she developing leg or hip issues like my previous dogs.

If a dog has some type of gait issue, I would recommend that they take the dog to a Rolfer™ before doing drugs or surgeries. Not that those things aren't appropriate at times, but only as a last resort. Unless there is a tumor or something similar that's causing the problem, I would definitely recommend a Rolfing series—I don't think it can do any harm. In Toni's case it did nothing but help her.

Toni is a very active dog. We do a two-mile walk each day, and on the weekend she is out running free when she's not running in the yard. Before I brought her in to Briah, I had taken her to the dog park and I could see that there was a hitch in her git-along. She was in pain, and I couldn't see where it was coming from. I even thought it might be hip displasia. But the Rolfing got rid of it and she is fine with it now.

She has a parallel, very proud gait without any limp. She is tracking really squarely with no variation at all—just very straight. She came from show dogs and her current gait is impressive to see.

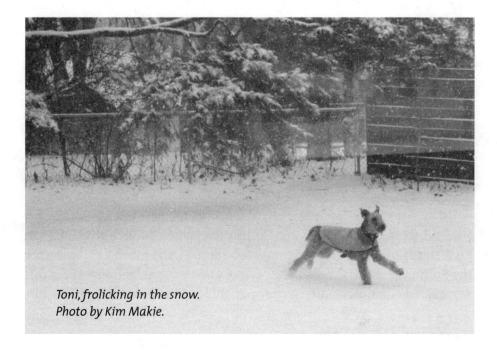

Toni, frolicking in the snow.
Photo by Kim Makie.

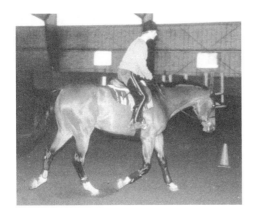
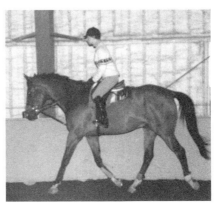
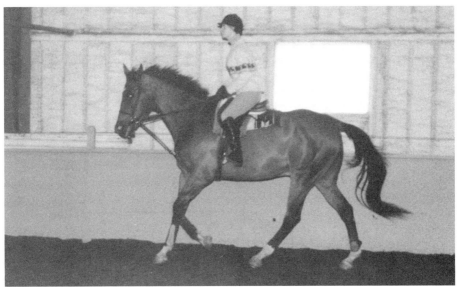

Andante Rising

Andante, a seven-year-old (eighteen-and-a-half hands tall), is a thoroughbred jumper. The rider is Lauren, a sixteen-year-old who aspires to be one of the ten best riders in the US. She came to be Rolfed because of her "poor posture/structure."

Top left. *Lauren and Andante in Dec. before Rolfing® SI. Note how collapsed Lauren looks and how far forward her neck and head are.* **Top right and bottom.** *Lauren after seven sessions and Andante after four Rolfing® SI sessions. In the after photos Lauren looks long, aligned, and energetic. Note the horse's gait and stride; now long, extended with beautiful lines and extension versus the short and contracted look before.*

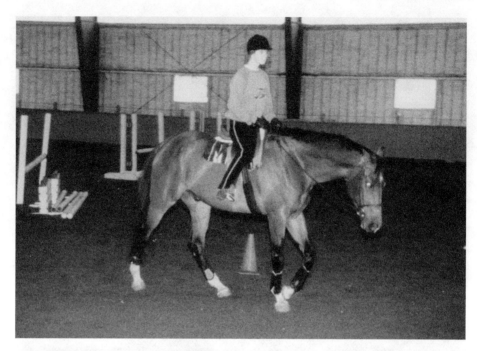

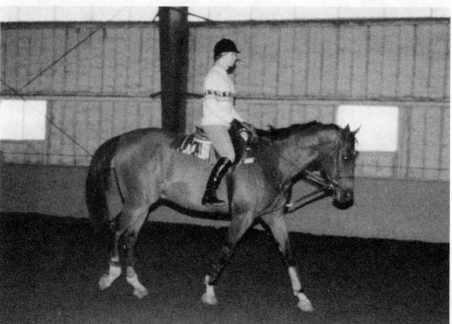

Top. *Another view of horse and rider before Rolfing® SI. Before Rolfing® SI, choppy, disconnected, stilted movements.* **Bottom.** *After session seven (rider) and session four (horse). Note structure change and elegance of movement. In the After photos and live performance they looked like dancers gliding through space. Quite beautiful to see!*

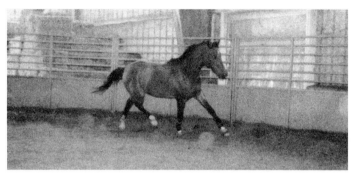

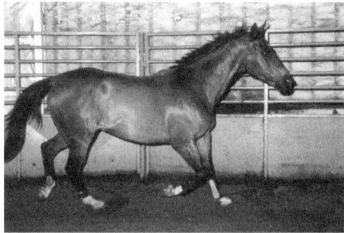

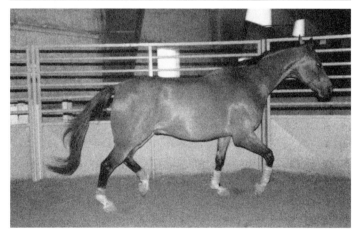

Top. *Andante in the round pen before Rolfing® SI. Note how stiff his legs are and how the right rear leg crosses the midline to a very medial and unbalanced position. The line of transmission and movement appears stiff and broken.* **Middle.** *Movement after four sessions. Note extension and lift in neck. Note distance of each leg— definite symmetry in gait.* **Bottom.** *Andante after 5 sessions. Length in torso and hind end is now present. Movement flows with ease and elegance. This is quite a transformed horse!*

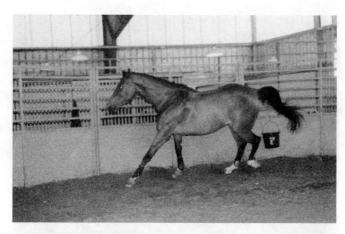

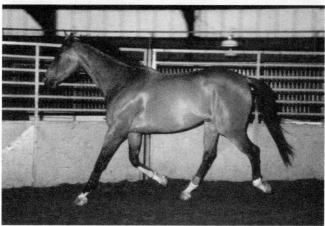

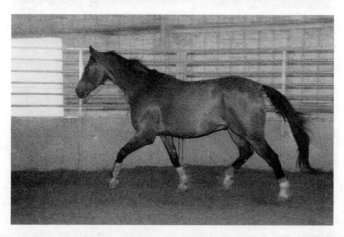

Top. *Before Rolfing® SI. Extension of left and right front legs is very straight and stiff, not conducive to a smooth, strong gait. This condition predisposes a jumping horse to many injuries as the impact from landing is hard and stiff.* **Middle.** *After four sessions. Note difference session five (bottom) brought to fruition.* **Bottom.** *After five sessions. Beautiful reach and extension with left front leg. Note left hind quarter and placement of left rear leg as it strikes the ground. Very square look and a true profile of hind quarter.*

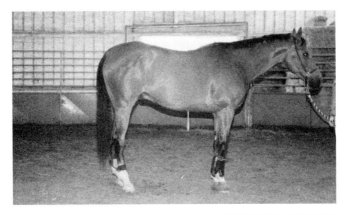

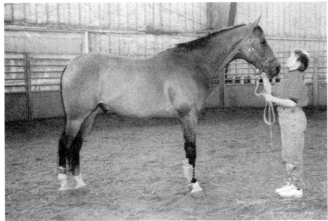

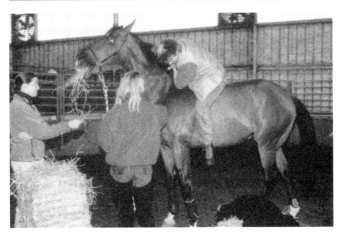

Top. *Before Rolfing® SI. Note front legs angle back; neck is proportionately too short for his structure, body of horse looks swayed; hind end is jammed, particularly the lumbar region.* **Middle.** *After five Rolfing® SI sessions. Note nice vertical alignment through front legs. Neck is longer and more uplifted. Body of horse looks longer and not swayed. Nice horizontal line is elongated and the right rear leg is not as twisted into the pelvis. Overall, Andante is longer, more filled out. There is a balance and symmetry of a much more regal jumper.* **Bottom.** *Working on the attachments of neck, shoulder, and legs.*

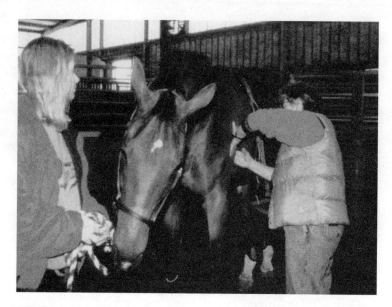

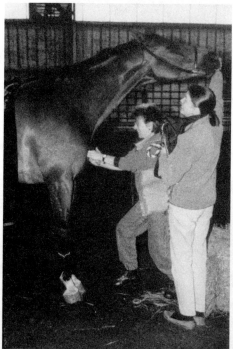

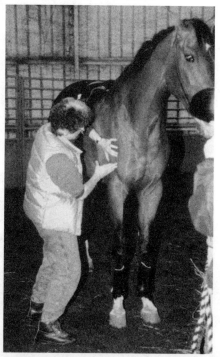

Top. *Note how Andante is twisting his neck and head. This is a wonderful response, very cooperative with my work. I'm working where the head and neck attach and he is instinctively pulling out of his restrictions.* **Bottom left.** *Beautiful and spontaneous stretching and extension of his neck and head. Andante knows he has a much longer neck in there.* **Bottom left.** *Notice glazed look in his eye. He is focused and listening yet very obviously in an altered state of consciousness.*

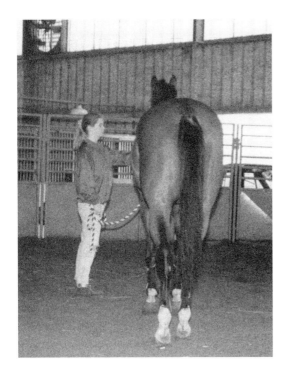

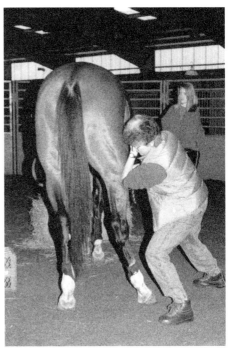

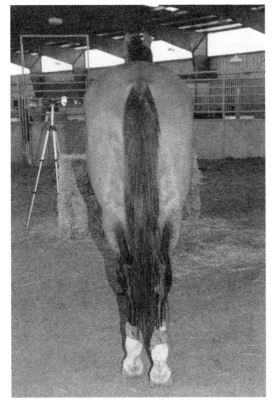

Top left. *Photo of rear before Rolfing® SI. Hind end is twisted hence showing much more of the left side than the right. Note placement of hind feet.* **Top right.** *First session. A priceless moment on film—Andante extending his rear right leg into me. I'm leaning into him with a lot of pressure. Natural cooperation and trust.* **Bottom.** *After five Rolfing® SI sessions. You can literally draw a vertical line up the middle of the tail and out of the top of the head. Note the side to side balance and symmetry. The hind end is now even. Before, one side was higher than the other.*

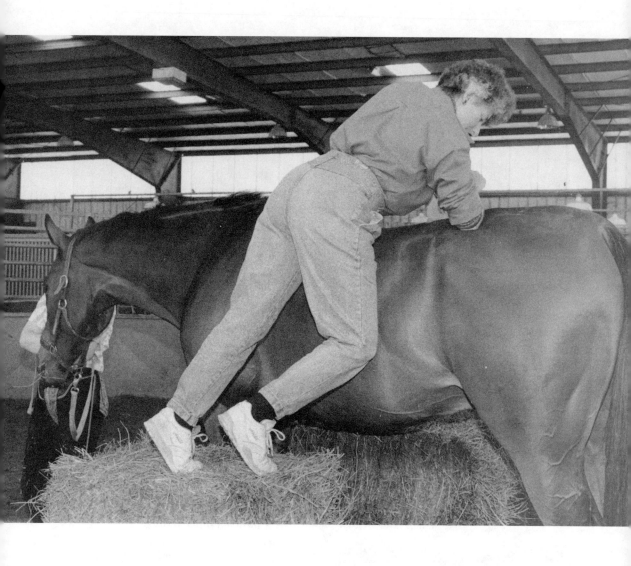

My last session with Andante. Both Andante and I working in harmony, exhibiting good form. Photos by Roy Inman.

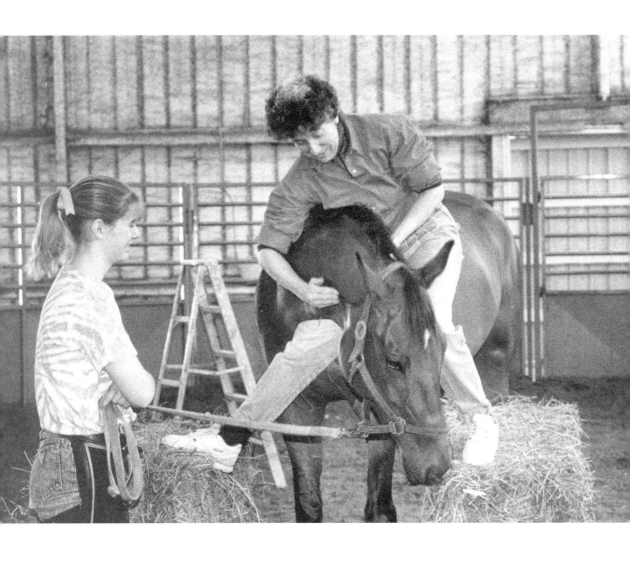

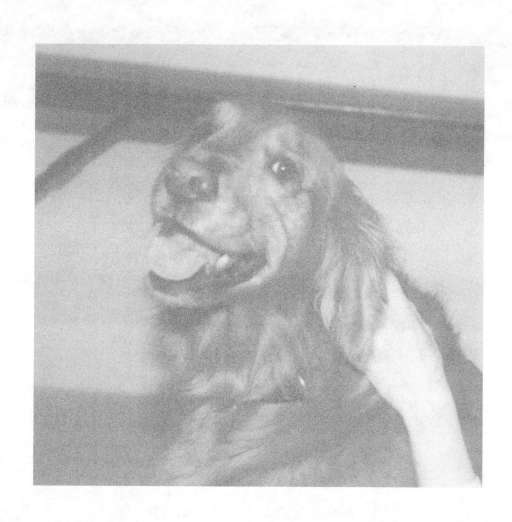

Going Out With Their Boots On

▶ *Body and mind are as two sides of the same coin, and so the results of working with the body reach into the emotional, behavioral, even spiritual life of the individual.*

▶ *Rolfing is a process of change. If we resist change, we experience pain.*

▶ *As a lighter, freer body comes into being, we can allow old patterns to disappear. Trust in our capacity to change grows, and we become sturdier.*

▶ *Some individuals may perceive their losing fight with gravity as a sharp pain in their back, others as the unflattering contour of their body, others as a constant fatigue, yet others as an unrelentingly threatening environment. Those over forty may call it old age. And yet, all these signals may be pointing to a single problem so prominent in their own structure, as well as others, that is has been ignored; they are off balance. They are at war with gravity.*

DR. IDA P. ROLF, from *Ida Rolf Talks about Rolfing and Physical Reality*, Rosemary Feitis, ed., Harper Row: NY; 1978

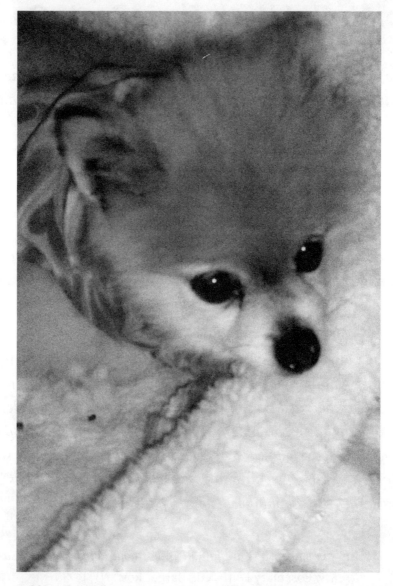

Babbles, the Bodhisattva—a treasure of the heart.

Babbles the Bodhisattva

Jeff Rutkowski, on his dog, Babbles

Our little Babbles came to us through a breeder in Texas after she gave birth to her one and only puppy. Her very small stature—only about five pounds—made birthing another puppy a risk to her health. Thus it was our fortune to welcome her into our family. Sometime at the end of 2008, Babbles developed a swollen breast. She was also twirling when she walked: taking a few steps and twirling, taking a few steps and twirling. We always thought that this was just a characteristic of her breed (Pomeranian), as they sometimes twirl when they are excited. It turned out that Babbles' twirling was a symptom of a larger issue.

Briah came to visit us at the end of February, 2009. She did two Rolfing® sessions on Babbles and intuitively suggested a homeopathic remedy. Right after the first session I noticed her form felt fuller when I held her, whereas before she had felt tight and somewhat wiry. After the second session I noticed Babbles felt like she had more structure to her. She also started walking in straight lines, no spinning, something we had never seen before. Another unexpected improvement was her nose. Ever since I can remember, Babbles' nose has been dry as bone, almost to the point of being chapped, but now it feels moist.

Before getting Rolfed Babbles had very little energy and would spend most of the day and night sleeping. She would only get up to come say hi every once in a while or ask for food. It was almost like she had given up. Now, she wants to spend time with us. Her eyes have more sparkle, she smiles more, she's bouncier, and just all around a happier dog. She has brought more light and energy to our home.

Briah told us that she feels like pets are "little bodhisattvas" who have come here to love and help us. Anyone who has ever felt down and had their dog come and paw at their leg or rest their head on their lap knows what I'm talking about. As a result of them being so hooked into us emotionally, as part of their communal pack mentality, they tend to absorb our emotional neuroses and general junk. I didn't know how true this was until after Briah had left.

Briah said she thought that Babbles's condition had to do with caretaking or mothering—Babbles licks incessantly almost like she's fawning over a puppy. We wondered if it had something to do with the one puppy she had birthed, but Briah suggested that it might have something to do with our family's emotional baggage. Three out of the five of us feel a very strong need to caretake in our relationships with others. We have a strong desire to make everybody feel okay, and make everything okay. My Dad has told me there are four types of people: analytical, driver, expressive, and amiable. You have never met a bigger family of amiable types. We want everyone to get along, and everything to be harmonious to such an extent that we sometimes stress ourselves over it. We're trying so hard to take care of everyone else we become alienated from our own needs. We're so focused on "mothering" everyone else, we forget to mother ourselves.

I came to realize this connection to Babbles' condition after I heard Briah talking to Babbles while she was working on her. She would tell her things like, "you're of such great consequence," "You're so important," and I realized I didn't feel comfortable saying those things out

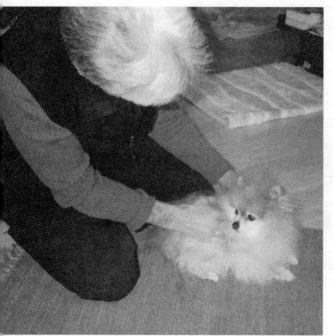

loud. If you can't say it to yourself you won't be able to say it to someone else and mean it.

Briah's encouragement also woke me up to Babbles as an aware little being. She knows what's going on and what people mean when they say something. Even small children who don't necessarily know what the topic of a conversation is can tell what the conversation feels like

My work with Babbles, a miniature Pomeranian, improved the quality of her last year of life.

from just a few words. Pets are the same. They know more than they let on. Animals are aware, conscious beings. They have physical, mental, emotional, and spiritual facets. Just because they don't speak our verbal language doesn't mean they don't have languages of their own. And it doesn't necessarily mean they don't understand our language. Words differ. Meaning is universal.

For instance, take Masaru Emoto's rice experiment: he took three jars of cooked rice and attached labels to two of them. One read: "Bakayarō" which translates as "you fool" or "you idiot" in Japanese. Another said "Arigatō" which means "thank you." The third jar was left blank. To each jar he said the words at least once a day while the blank jar was ignored. The "thank you" rice fermented, turning a cream color while the "you idiot" rice turned black. The most astounding thing is not just that the ignored rice also turned black, but that it turned black much faster than the "you idiot" rice. This shows us that the quality of our words is important, but even more important is just giving attention in the first place (i.e., acknowledging the existence of whatever we are paying attention to).

This experiment has been replicated all over the world in many languages producing similar results showing that it really is the language of the heart (meaning) that matters most. I think this is especially important in relation to our animals. Just like when you hear "I love you" from somebody and can immediately know whether it is just a perfunctory statement or arising from actual felt love, animals know when we're paying them genuine attention, or just "going through the motions." I don't think they take it personally though. If you've ever pet a cat, you know that they're just happy to have you petting them. Same with our dogs, they're just happy to have us around.

Babbles still has problems, but she's worlds better than she was before the Rolfing. We all have a new appreciation for our amazing dog as a multi-faceted aware little being. We show her more attention and love now, and the growth of our awareness is the biggest gift we could have received from the experience—the treasures of the heart really are the most important. I feel Rolfing is a key facilitator in the release of old patterns—both physical and emotional—but it's always a joint venture between the Rolfer™ and the client. We owners are as much clients as the pets themselves. We have to find our center, our line, our meaning and direction, for ourselves as much as for our little bodhisattvas.

Aging Into Liveliness and Love

Beverly MacDougall, on her dog, Mac

Mac is a fourteen-year-old toy poodle. He has always had difficulty with dislocating joints, something inherent to many poodles. As he aged he began to not care for walking because he would often go lame in his right hind leg. His walk became more of a painful hobble as the years went by.

A year ago he jumped off of a chair and began screeching very loudly. His right shoulder had crossed over his chest and I was afraid he'd dislocated it. We took him to the vet and had to wait awhile to get in. As we were waiting Mac calmed down, and then wanted to get down on the floor. Dave put him down and Mac was soon walking with no limp at all. So it had cleared itself. We had noticed earlier that it felt like a tendon had crossed to the front of his leg that should have been at the back. It pulled for awhile and then just settled back down in the right place. This happened a couple of times after that first incident and we didn't do anything about it because we knew it would clear.

Around that time I was seeing Briah for Rolfing® myself, and we decided to see what it could do for Mac. When I took him in to Briah for the first session, I didn't know how he would react to someone handling him the way she would with the Rolfing, but he just settled right down, and seemed to say, "okay, go ahead." He talked to her a couple of times, but made no attempt to get away or hide. It surprised me that he knew intuitively what he needed and would turn over after Briah had worked on one side long enough without her asking him to. I didn't know what to expect, but I didn't expect that.

During the second session he was a little less agreeable—not angry or upset, but trying to walk away when she was working on his hips.

It hadn't seemed to bother him during the first session and he even enjoyed it. But during the second session it was as if he felt, "I don't think I need this!" But he did, and it's made a difference in him. He's moving better and he's more coordinated with his body's motions. He's more aware of what goes where, when.

Mac is very different now after his two Rolfing sessions. He doesn't feel quite as bony—there's more muscle on him. He's a very small dog, only 3.2 pounds, but he feels more solid now. When I run my hand over his ribs there's more tissue over them and he's cuddlier than he used to be. He is now standing up on his hind legs when he wants something like he used to when he was a puppy. He doesn't limp and hasn't had any more problems with his shoulder. He seems more relaxed. He's always been fairly calm but he's more inside his body. When I hold him from the front by his front paws now, instead of his right side crunching up, it falls down naturally. Whatever had been pulling that right side short has let go.

Sometime after the second session Briah came to our house to receive a session from me. (I do Frequencies of Brilliance work.) Mac was at the door. Briah came in and since he doesn't see very well, he didn't know who she was for a minute. After she spoke to him and bent down, his tail just started to go in a circle! He was so happy. Licking and kissing and just really, really, really happy to see her. He probably thought that she was coming to work on him! Rolfing has made a big difference in him, and I know that he appreciated it because he didn't try to get away from her—he went right to her once he smelled her and recognition set in. All the expressions of liking and wanting to be close that he could give, he gave to her. So it was good!

His eating and elimination have changed too. He's not trying to scarf food as much as he did, and I don't know if it's because we're feeding him a little more or if he recognizes that he doesn't need as much (or maybe he just doesn't see it). He used to be a great scarfer of food. He looked for little bits of anything, and if you dropped something on the floor it was gone faster than a speeding bullet.

He's eating a little bit more because the vet said we could feed him more now. Instead of having a bowel movement once a day, he's having a bowel movement every time he goes out, which is good. As for urine, that hasn't really changed. He now comes up to me with a certain look that I recognize, so I'll head toward the door. He runs right after me and goes out. So he's more in tune with his own body. It's nice.

At fourteen and a half, he's blind and deaf, so his only sense for orientation has been smell. I think his sight has come back a little though because during the day he will go outside, and up and down the stairs better than he used to. He seems to be walking with more confidence and not walking into walls anymore. In the dark he is tentative but he can still make his way. Before the Rolfing, he would walk into the walls, and in the dark he would just stand and not know where to go because he couldn't see what was in front of him. He's more sure footed now, and more active.

He seems more peaceful, too. I used to look at him and wonder if I had to buy more dog food because he just didn't seem to have a desire to live. He didn't move much. He didn't get excited about bananas or peanut butter (his favorite treats). He just sort of dragged around. He could get himself to places he wanted to go but not in the easy, puppy-like way that he does now. He's almost like a puppy again in the way he moves.

I really didn't know how long I'd have him with me. I took him to the vet once because I wanted to know if Mac was happy without being able to see or hear. He used to back away from us when we walked up to touch him because he couldn't hear us coming. He's not doing that now, and he's definitely rediscovered peanut butter.

To people who have older dogs like Mac, I'd say that Rolfing is very well worth it. If you want your dog to feel good physically again, this is

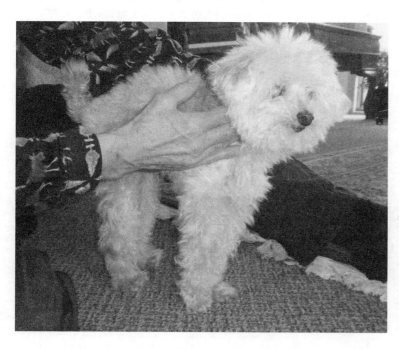

Mac, a fourteen-year-old toy poodle, who was failing in life reminded me that Rolfing® SI can affect animals at any stage of life or condition in a positive way.

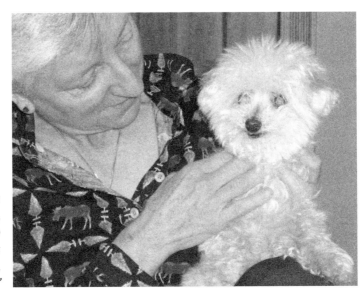

Beverly, Mac's owner, says, "After these two sessions Mac's a different dog. He's more dog!"

definitely going to help. It will loosen up the tissues so they can get back to where they belong, not where they've gone over a lifetime. Their bodies get supported again and they move freely. You'll like the result. You'll see a dog that's functioning with more ease, calmer and more peaceful. Mac doesn't even squawk too much in his bath now—he never liked his bath, but now he seems to say, "Okay, bathe me!"

I can't tell you all the ways that Mac is different now, but I know he's not the same dog. He's more like he was when he was younger, but now he's more connected to us. He wants to be around us. When we come back to the house, if one of us comes in first and greets him, he starts whimpering and looking for the other one. He wants both of us here. He's just a little softie, and he talks.

I don't know a lot about other animals, I just know about the two dogs I've had, and I really wish that I had known about Rolfing when my dog, Kelsey, was still alive. I think he would have lived a longer, happier life than he did. I wouldn't have ever thought of Rolfing for a dog, even though I get Rolfing for myself. But why not Rolf a pet if the pet is in distress? It's going to make a difference.

After the first session of Rolfing Briah did with me, my whole posture changed. I stood up straighter and my stomach fell back. My posture continued to change and lengthen for awhile. I haven't measured myself but I'm sure I'm a couple of inches taller. It was what I needed to do to open up to where I should be, instead of where a lifetime of working and being a mother and hauling kids around has put me. I'm a different person, and Mac's a different dog. He's *more dog.*

Because I'd felt like he was not going to be around much longer, like I could lose him any day, I had started to protect myself from that coming pain. I cut myself off from him. I got angry at him. I didn't want him around. I didn't want to go through that pain again. But now I don't worry about him and whether he might go lame. I don't worry if he jumps thinking he might screw up his shoulder. I don't worry about him, I just love him now. I can open back up to him even more than I ever did. With the Rolfing have come changes in me and changes in Mac. I like just holding him; I never used to. I like just holding him and petting him. He's been opened up to me in a whole new way, and there's more connection between the two of us. He was always Dave's dog, and now he's both of ours. We're more tuned in to each other than we ever were.

Mac is fourteen and otherwise healthy, but I know that he' not going to be around a whole lot longer. I do know that he's going to meet his end in a better state of physicality and mind than he would have without Rolfing. And we'll be easier too because he's a calmer, more peaceful, happier dog, wanting company, and enjoying his sleeps. He wants to be around us instead of crawling into his cage or cuddling up in the corner of the couch when we're somewhere else. He's looking for us now, he's wanting to be with us, so that's really nice, and I've fallen in love with my dog again.

Aging and Pain Management

Tanya Sayles, on her golden retriever, Isabella

Izzy first saw Briah about seven years ago after I had a Rolfing® session from Briah. I completed the ten-series with her, and when Briah mentioned she worked with dogs, I decided to get a session for Izzy, even though she is only four years old and doesn't have issues. But Izzy loved it.

She did very well for about six years, until three months ago when she started limping. We brought her to the vet who found that she had hip dysplasia. They said this was common with golden retrievers, especially older dogs. Izzy was now ten years old. They gave her anti-inflammatory painkillers and that seemed to do the trick. She seemed fine and her personality improved; she had been a little depressed before with the hip dysplasia and pain.

Then it reoccurred a month ago—she could barely walk and seemed very depressed. Trying to go to the bathroom was difficult, and she was going downhill rapidly. Then I remembered Briah, so I called and Briah got us in right away. Izzy had one session and she seemed better, but she just still acted very depressed, and it was hard to walk. I took her to the vet because the next Rolfing session wasn't for another week and a half and I wanted to get Izzy some help before that. They gave her another round of painkillers and antibiotics because she had an infection.

Izzy had her second session with Briah and she seemed a lot better afterward. I think that the Rolfing was starting to kick in and the pain was being relieved with the painkillers. Her personality started to perk up and the tail would wag and her old gait was coming back. She has a strong wiggle and it was good to see that movement return. After her third session, we were really noticing a huge, huge difference. She had her full gait back, she was happy, the infection cleared up, and I reduced her pain meds.

She remembered Briah when I took her back six years later; she went right to her with a big smile. This is a very friendly dog to begin with, but she knew what Briah was about, and it was like, "Oh, I'm going to get body-work!" She would lay down and show Briah where it hurt. She would lay on her side and have the hip up that hurt so Briah would know where to start. She didn't resist the work at all—she really enjoys it. In fact I'm sure she was trying to say: "Bring me to Briah, don't give me these pills!"

Both her personality and mobility have greatly improved. I think she is aging now—her fur is getting more coarse like it does in an aging dog. I think that if she was younger some things could hold longer. Because she is an older dog, when she plays or exercises too much, the dysplasia and pain reoccur. If it's not too bad I give her the homeopathic remedies, Arnica and Rhus Tox. When those don't do the trick, I give her a few anti-inflammatory painkillers.

Briah and I talked about how she's an older dog and if she could get Rolfing on a regular basis, that would be perfect. But not everybody has that kind of resources. When a dog gets older sometimes the best thing to do is to make them as comfortable as possible because you can't com-

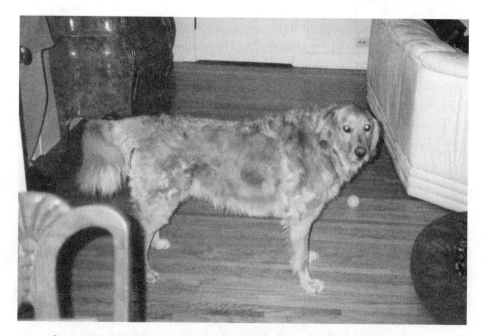

Izzy, a four-year-old golden retriever after her first Rolfing® SI session looking stretched out, well aligned and content.

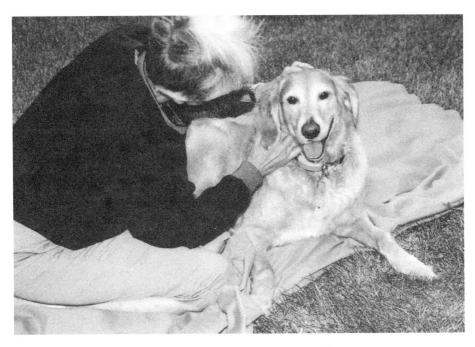

At age ten Izzy was brought back to work with me around her aging issues. Izzy was experiencing lack of mobility and increased pain. The process was comforting for both Izzy and her family.

pletely take away whatever they're suffering from. As people or animals get older you can only do so much, and it becomes more about helping them deal with their pain. Instead of being able to completely alleviate it, you can help them suffer less.

I think the early Rolfing sessions when she was four years old made a difference for the ensuing six years. She didn't see Briah again until she was ten. I think whatever people can do when their dogs are younger is the best way to help a dog age, because like Briah said, these conditions are things that we've had for a long time.

For example, dogs have a hip dysplasia issue when they're young, but the symptoms show up or get worse with age. Izzy probably had it as a young dog, but the symptoms just didn't come up until later. Perhaps they were less severe because of the early Rolfing. If people knew more about Rolfing they wouldn't have to resort to surgery so often. People with older dogs are just trying to make them comfortable. It's not about healing them completely, and many owners don't want to put an older dog through a major surgery—they just couldn't handle it. Rolfing is a nice option to help with the pain management.

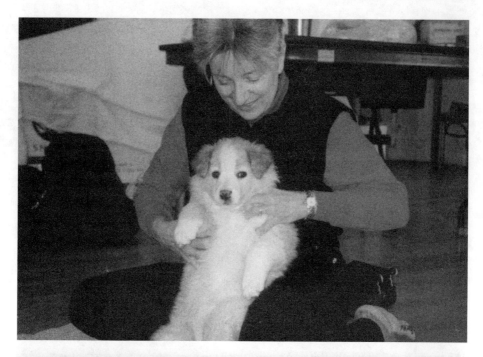

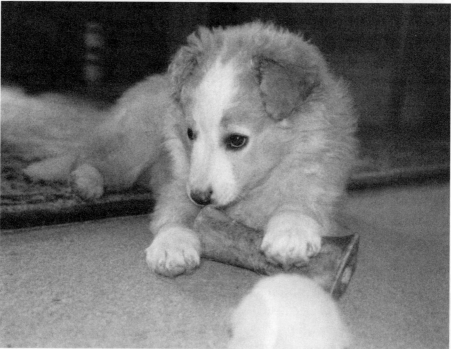

Top. *Cassie, a two-and-a-half-month-old English shepherd receiving a Rolfing® SI session as preventive care.* **Bottom.** *No bone seems too big for Cassie to handle! Photos by Valerie Ohanian.*

Prevention: The Dog Owner's Best Friend

Valerie Ohanian, on homeopathy, Rolfing® SI, and her dog, Cassie.
Valerie is the cofounder and Dean of the Northwestern Academy
of Homeopathy, in Minneapolis, Minnesota.

Cassie is an English shepherd who is now seven years old, and she had a Rolfing session two days after we brought her home from the farm.

The English shepherd is an unusual breed in this country. They are dogs that are born to run, they're fairly bossy, and Cassie was a very dominant puppy. We brought her home from the barn and she was completely out of control, so she had a Rolfing session in which Briah did, I assume, the usual healthy puppy Rolfing session. Cassie was eight weeks old at the time. I was particularly interested in what Rolfing would do for her because this breed had developed hip dysplasia in the last few years. Cassie's parents didn't have it, but there were no guarantees that Cassie wouldn't, so prevention seemed to be the best measure. I'm happy to say Cassie's hips have been great. She runs very freely and can run for hours if given the opportunity.

What I noticed after her Rolfing session was that she seemed to settle into herself. Rolfing didn't change her personality; she is still a dominant, bossy dog, but she went from being hyperactive to more normal and more grounded. For example, before she was Rolfed, she would come to a class I was teaching and would be so crazed that she just ran in circles. Just an hour after the Rolfing session, she went into the class and politely greeted each person individually, then went and sat down—a night and day difference. So those are the main changes we've seen.

I don't really remember Cassie having any injuries; when I think about her, what I think about is how healthy she has been. She has not had a sick day in her life. If somebody she loves is missing for a bit, she can get a little sad, but is always ready to go and play, and she has been very healthy and very strong.

Improved Function for Animals with Structural Issues

Over the years, I've referred other people with animals who were having some issues, but unfortunately I think too many people wait to take their animals to get Rolfing until they are on their last legs. One of my neighbors had a huge German shepherd, a 145-pound dog, whose hips were so bad that he couldn't get outside. He had a few Rolfing sessions with Briah and those sessions probably gave him another year or year and a half. He went from not being able to walk to being able to walk to some degree. If he'd come five years earlier, I think it would have made an even bigger difference.

Another dog I referred was a border collie with debilitating arthritis, and her family waited until she was eleven or twelve before they brought her in for Rolfing work. It helped her arthritis enough so that she could move around again, and she is ready to come back for more. Again, the concern I have is that her people should have brought her back six months ago. People don't think of Rofing as readily as they should, but it is a great treatment for animals. I've been reading lately about how acupuncture for dogs is taking off, and acupuncture certainly can help, but animal acupuncture is much more treatment-intensive than Rolfing. They see the dogs every week for six weeks, and then every other week for nine to twelve weeks.

Acupuncture can relieve pain, but for a structural problem like hip dysplasia, which is one of the more endemic issues in animals these days, there is nothing really except Rolfing that will help it, in my experience. Briah has data about that and data speaks for itself, but what speaks more potently is seeing an animal who can't move freely be able to get up and start moving. That's what really makes a difference. I don't know that there is a medium or large breed purebred dog in this country anymore that's not subject to hip or shoulder dysplasia.

Cassie's breed, the English shepherd, is not an AKC recognized breed so it hasn't been overbred, but even with twenty careful breeders in the country, these issues are starting to show up. Anybody who buys a purebred dog with the potential for dysplasia should get that dog Rolfed when it's a puppy before the structure is too well set, rather than waiting until the very end of life. That's what makes sense to me. In my experience, animals respond very quickly to this kind of therapy.

Without Resistance, Change Happens Quickly

In my practice as a homeopath, I have referred many people for Rolfing work and I've had the work myself. Rolfing is a very effective and potent therapy, and in humans, myself included, we all have emotional issues and stresses that we hold in our bodies from doing more than we can do in the world. Rolfers™ have to get through these kinds of emotional blocks in humans. But, at least in my experience with dogs, they don't have those blocks for the most part, so the work gets in without much resistance at all. Where it may take twenty sessions with a human to get the requested and required change, with a dog it can happen in three to five sessions at most.

While Rolfing is very effective for people, in animals it's just more of a direct transfer. Cassie is a dog who is very sensitive to being touched in a negative way. She can bark and growl and snap, but with Briah, she is aware that something is going on. She's a restless dog so she doesn't really like sitting, but she works with Briah in the best way she can. She will immediately lie down and turn over on her back. When she's receiving a session she's accepting the work. Her face is smoothed out. She is paying attention to what's happening in her body, and animals can do that in a way that humans don't find easy to do. Even though one might think an animal would be more resistant to the work, I think it's just the opposite. Change occurs much faster. They're more easily connected with their bodies and they depend on them more in a certain way than we do.

When a puppy gets Rolfing at the beginning of life before their problems have set in, it takes one session; two if the animal has more difficult breeding or is bigger. If it's a puppy, Briah can accomplish everything in one session and that's such a small investment for a lifetime of an aligned structure. Not only is that structure important for hips and shoulders, but a Rolfed dog is a healthier dog in general. They have better digestion which is a key to a dog's health. What you feed a dog is vitally important, but again, the small investment of one Rolfing session in puppyhood can make a huge difference in the nutritional processing of a dog and its health. I don't think Rolfed puppies get chronically ill. If one inherits a dog, or gets a one-year old or two-year-old, it's still not too late. Prevention in this way is worth all the treatment otherwise needed when a dog is arthritic, stuck, tight, or traumatized.

I also refer people to get Rolfing for their dogs after any kind of accident, even an accident where they haven't been badly hurt such as slipping on the ice, taking a bad fall, being in a fight. Even a friendly fight with another dog can throw things off. If the animal doesn't seem to have anything wrong but doesn't seem quite right, it is also worth considering getting work done at that point.

How Rolfing SI and Homeopathy Work Together to Address Chronic Conditions

People tend to bring animals to homeopaths when the animals have a chronic illness that either cannot be treated by conventional veterinary work, or it would be way too expensive and invasive. What we as homeopaths do is try and raise the animal's vitality to the highest level through giving the remedy that best matches that animal's nature. Rolfing is a complement to homeopathy in that Rolfing raises vitality as well through direct connection with tissues. Remedies affect the energy directly, Rolfing affects the tissues directly, and the combination raises energy and really balances out the individual animal.

Homeopathy can be helpful in structural issues when the issues are chronic. They can be chronic to that particular animal, chronic joint issues like shoulder joint issues, chronic in terms of that animal's history, or even chronic in the knowledge of the breed. Where Rolfing will realign the structure, homeopathy can actually have an impact on how the inherited illnesses affect the individual dog, and so working with both modalities together is an excellent way to get increased health.

Cassie has a limp that is noticeable but it doesn't impede her. My concern is that most people seeing a limp like this would just let the animal be. That's a good idea, better to let her be than take her to a vet and get anti-inflammatory drugs or things that would upset her system. But when something as direct as Rolfing could help, it just makes more sense to think of Rolfing in these kind of situations. If there is some kind of strain or minor upset, dogs let us know how they feel. Even if they don't whine and complain like we humans, we can see it.

Rolfing SI as Preventive Care

In terms of chronic health problems, that initial Rolfing session in puppyhood or at least in the first year, can make a difference between having an animal that's healthy in all ways and one that is chronically ill. Not only does the Rolfing set up the animal for a strong structure, it impacts the internal organs. Dogs age much more quickly than humans—in one year a dog ages the equivalent of seven human years. If there is a possibility of an organ problem such as liver cancer, lung problems, or lung tumors, having that dog Rolfed as a pup may very well eliminate or at least postpone the development of those problems until very old age. It used to be that dogs typically lived to the age of ten to fourteen without health problems. Now it is rare to see purebreds hit that ten or twelve-year mark without some kind of health issue, and I think Rolfing can help prevent those issues from occurring.

The Rolfing process can also soothe a dog's nervous system. So many dogs these days have to be left home alone, and dogs by nature are meant to be in company. They're meant to be in packs with other dogs, other animals, or with humans. When they're not, they can go kind of nuts—so much so that many vets are putting dogs on anti-anxiety and antidepressant medicines. Prozac for dogs is not a joke, it's a real thing. Rolfing impacts the nervous system and can help dogs be much more settled in themselves than they might ordinarily be, especially breeds that have been bred to work. Working dogs tend to be more hyper if not worked every day.

Even dogs that are highly strung like terriers, who have quite wound-up nervous systems, can be settled down. It might take several sessions, but Cassie's nervous system benefited from one session. Better for the dog to be Rolfed than to take medicines which are hard on its inner organs and can set it up to have more health problems down the road. Nobody wants a dog destroying their house, and doggie daycare can be very expensive. It's better to help the dog in some positive ways and have a happy dog at home watching the squirrels and birds.

Allergy problems can also be helped by Rolfing because it helps move the energy through the tissues. Allergies occur where energy is stuck or dead, and Rolfing will increase circulation on all those levels which will help improve allergies.

Vaccinations are another troublesome problem that Rolfing has been very effective with. Now, there is a great deal of controversy about vaccines for animals, but the fact is dogs have to be vaccinated to go to dog training, to get on airplanes, or to cross state lines, so even owners who don't really want to vaccinate their dogs end up having to do so. In some animals, vaccination can cause skin allergy, joint and muscle problems, and Rolfing is even beneficial for a post-vaccinated dog.

Another dog I referred to Rolfing, and also to homeopathy, was a Boxer who was very well taken care of, its owner's best friend, a very sensitive, gentle dog who had cancer that was going to take the dog's life. Its owner made a decision not to put the dog through invasive, expensive chemotherapy and radiation, and instead turned to Rolfing and homeopathy. The result is that the dog is now cancer-free and very healthy. I can't underscore how quickly dogs respond to appropriate treatment, and in this case the combination of treatments was necessary. The homeopathy raised the vital force of the animal, the Rolfing helped free the animal, and it was a far less expensive endeavor than having the medical treatments done. These treatments didn't hurt the dog, didn't cause pain, didn't cause disruption. They are very gentle, easy treatments. So the dog really came back to herself.

There is not a disease out there that the combination of good immune-enhancing treatments can't impact, those treatments being Rolfing and homeopathy. Interestingly, many diseases that dogs are getting these days are autoimmune diseases, for which the combination of Rolfing and homeopathy is excellent.

The diseases I'm seeing most commonly include the connective tissue diseases, cancers of all kinds, skin diseases that are immune related, severe allergies, eczema in dogs, psoriasis, and issues that have come from too much inbreeding. The allopathic interventions for these diseases are heavy doses of cortisones which shut down the immune system. Rolfing and homeopathy actually support the immune system. They will strengthen underactive immune systems and balance overactive immune systems. They will increase the body's ability to seek out and destroy cancer cells. It's not so easy to treat an animal for cancer with homeopathy and Rolfing if the animal has had invasive treatment like surgery, radiation and chemotherapy. But if the animal has not had any of those things, which fortunately most animals haven't because their owners won't put them through it, they can easily be helped.

Homeopathic vets have a success rate of about 80 percent, and when you add in Rolfing, I think that rate goes up to a much higher percentage and a longer lasting cure.

Treating Hip Dysplasia with Rolfing SI, or Delaying Symptom Onset

Hip dysplasia is something that Rolfing has a big impact on. When you look at the alternatives, even other alternative therapies, acupuncture can relieve pain but can't improve the quality of the structure; homeopathy can relieve pain but again, it's not going to change the structure. Conventional medicine provides surgery which sometimes corrects, sometimes doesn't, has a very painful recovery for the animals, and is very expensive. You're looking at $5,000 or more for a surgery that may or may not make a difference, and if it does make a difference, it's small. A conscientious vet will not promise this as a cure-all.

For dogs where surgery isn't possible, steroid injections or oral steroids are the treatment of choice. These can again relieve pain, but—unlike acupuncture or homeopathy—cause damage to the internal structure. Dogs being given steroids are more likely to develop connective tissue problems, joint dysfunctions, or arthritis at an early age. We know that even with humans, high doses of steroids promote arthritic development. Dogs, with their very quick aging, are going to develop those conditions much faster. They're going to set in much more quickly and be much more debilitating than they are for a human.

These are all good reasons to treat hip dysplasia with Rolfing, or get animals Rolfed before they develop any signs or symptoms. With any breed that has a likelihood of hip dysplasia, you might as well just assume your dog is going to get it. It's not an if, it's more like a when. If you get the dog treated, they are not going to have bad hips starting at the age of twelve when they are also getting arthritic and debilitated before their years. Rolfing not only can prevent problems like that, but it can give us the thing we want most of all for our animals which is to have happy, long lives.

In summary, Rolfing is greatly beneficial for dogs, both in terms of prevention and cure. There are few modalities that can boast that kind of success. With regard to problems or illnesses that are inherent in a breed, everything from hip and shoulder dysplasia, cancers and autoimmune issues, to arthritis and tightness, Rolfing can help prevent all those conditions. For both immune health and structural health, there is not a better modality for animals.

A Second Wind for Jessie

A twelve-year-old collie, Jessie's owners had taken her to the vet because she was limping—she would place her weight down carefully as the pads of her feet were quite tender. The vet diagnosed her problem as a combination of old age and arthritis. After only one Rolfing® session, even the neighbors remarked that Jessie was running around like her old self.

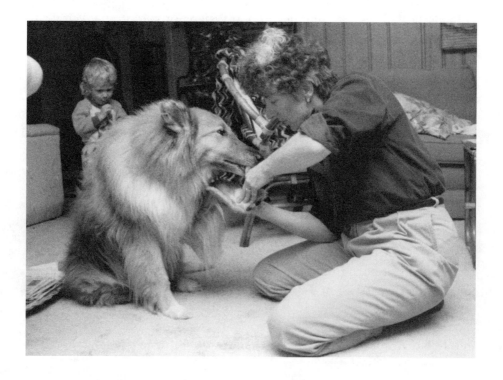

The Good Life

Morgan Rutherford reminisces about Briah's dog, Shelby

Briah asked me to reflect on my experiences with Shelby twelve years ago and my remembrance of that early relationship is much the same now as it was then. Most interesting to note, however, are the changes the passage of time can bring to any relationship, and how we choose to learn from our experiences.

Since my reflection twelve years ago, Shelby has passed away. She was truly the perfect dog, and I still find myself thinking of her from time to time and missing her very much. She was an absolutely beautiful presence in my life, and I feel my connection to her has led me to understand certain aspects of Rolfing® and its effects, and to more deeply appreciate how Rolfing can affect an animal just as much as, if not more, than a human being.

I first met Shelby when my mother brought me along for a Rolfing session she had scheduled for herself with Briah. When the door opened I was immediately greeted by a beautiful golden retriever, followed closely by Briah, smiling and ushering us into the room beyond. I remember liking Briah and the room, but most of all I remember instantly loving Shelby so much that I begged my mother to take me with her to every appointment. During one of those appointments Briah informed me she had done Rolfing sessions on many animals. She showed me impressive pictures of herself working with mountain lions, eagles, stallions, and even Shelby.

Looking back on this, I see how obvious it was that Shelby had had Rolfing work. She was unlike any dog I have ever met. I have known many golden retrievers over the years, and while all of them were friendly, good-natured and well-behaved, Shelby had a depth that I can only describe as human. Rolfing gave Shelby much more than good form. She was more aware of her surroundings than other dogs. The layers of Shelby's being were opened up; it seemed to me that this work had allowed her to become who she was really meant to be. She had more depth and knowing than many humans, and was able to express herself with great clarity.

At our first meeting, I sat down on the floor to pet Shelby, and she sat down right in my lap despite her size. This became our routine; often we would sit on the floor while I petted and massaged her for the entire session. She would know just when my legs must be getting numb and roll onto her back so I could scratch her underside.

Shelby had certain toys that she associated with certain people. She always brought out a little knobby squeak-toy for me. This was purely for her own enjoyment, although she would often set the toy gingerly in my lap, a drool-covered offering.

After my mother had finished her series of ten sessions, it was my turn for a Rolfing series. I remember Shelby being close by my side as we began. As we started the series, Briah took photographs of me as a "before" reference. We had to send Shelby out of the room with my mother because Shelby was glued to my hip in every shot. It is interesting now to think back and realize just how much Shelby is ingrained in my memory

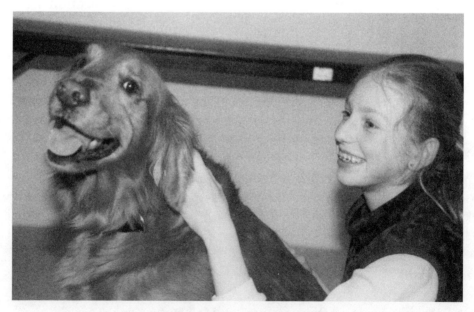

Morgan playing with my (Rolfing® SI assistant) Shelby. Morgan continues to be deeply influenced by the memory of Shelby and appreciative of the times they shared together.

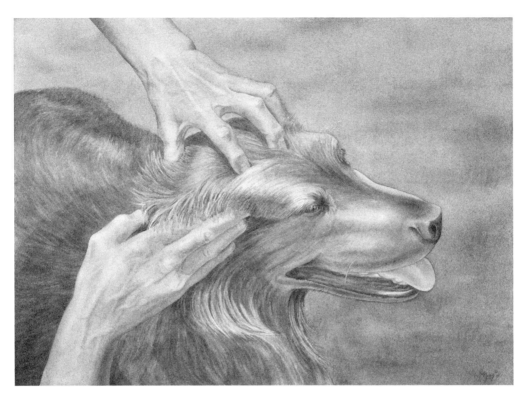

This painting of me working on Shelby was commissioned over 10 years ago and represents Shelby's love of Rolfing® SI and my love of working with animals. Painting by Carol Gray.

and experience with Rolfing. I think Shelby picked up on the energy in the room and did her part to help the client.

I remember Shelby "talking" to me many times while I lay on the Rolfing table. I had the clear impression that she was explaining something to me at length. Looking back, I think she felt she knew how to help me work through my own Rolfing sessions, offering encouragement. If Briah began to work in an area that was uncomfortable, Shelby would suddenly be at my side. I would feel her head slip under my hand, and she would rest her face there, inches from me, clearly aware she had a comforting effect.

Shelby and I became connected on a deep level. Briah was aware of this, and often had me over to visit Shelby. I remember when Briah asked me to dog-sit for her. Taking Shelby on walks, I got to see her in action and how obvious it was that she had been Rolfed. She was so responsive to me as we walked, paying attention to my movements and reacting accordingly. She was calm and graceful as we walked, and caught the eye of the people we passed.

Now, as a college student, one of my favorite jobs has been dog-sitting for various people, and I still believe Shelby was the easiest and most enjoyable dog to walk with. So many people try everything to get their dog to be a "good walker," often using choke chains, harnesses and muzzles. Shelby's ability to be a good walker came from having a good foundation, both physically and mentally.

Having had time for my own Rolfing sessions to integrate and grow with me, I realize that Rolfing does not simply align the physical body, it also connects the mind and body. Walking with Shelby it was clear that she not only had a good physical ability to stay in line and keep an even gait, but also the mental capacity to control herself. She could see what I wanted, and knew what her body had to do to obey the commands.

All of this is not to say that Rolfing took any dog-like qualities from her. Shelby was a very playful, friendly dog who still found her way into trouble and mischief. She still needed to be played with, monitored, and reprimanded. Rolfing may have had a profound effect on Shelby, but it did not make her any less of a golden retriever. If anything, Rolfing enhanced her ability to simply be a dog.

Photo Gallery of Briah's Animal Clients

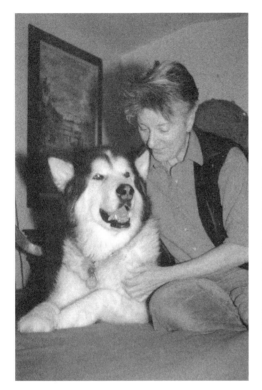
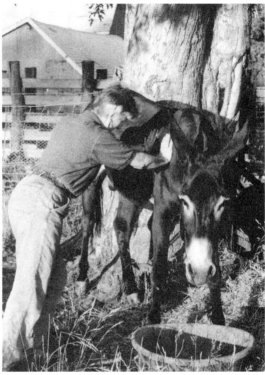
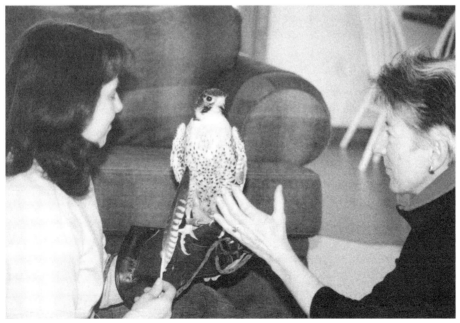

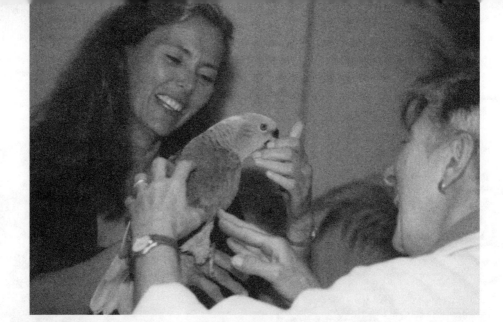
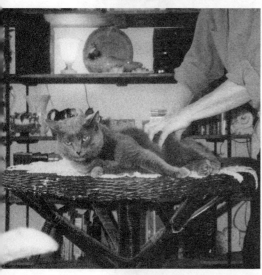
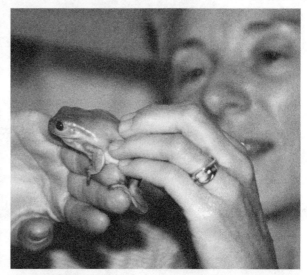
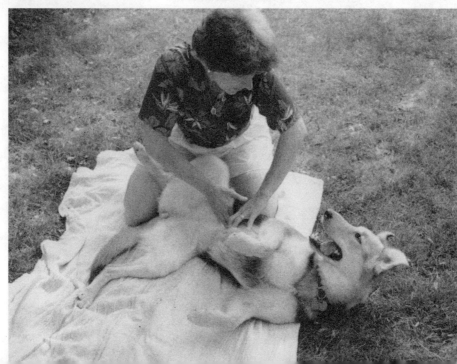

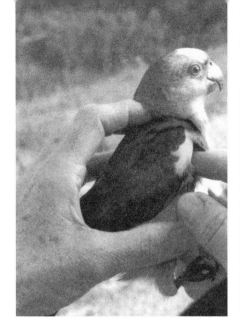
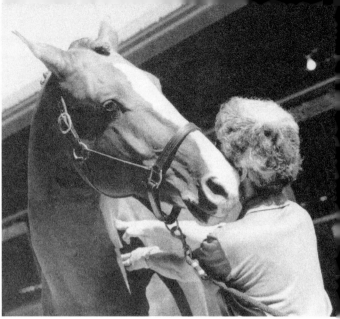
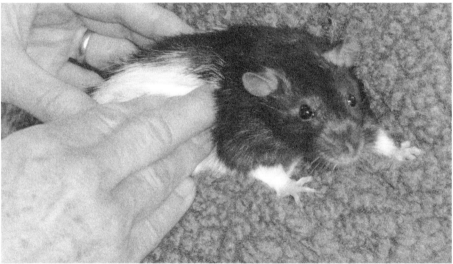
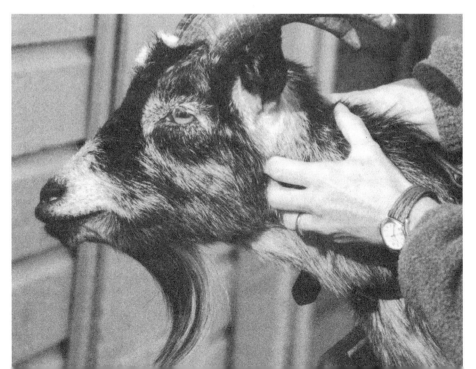

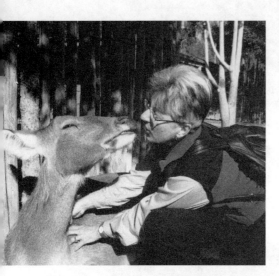

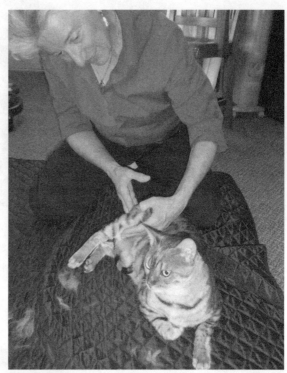

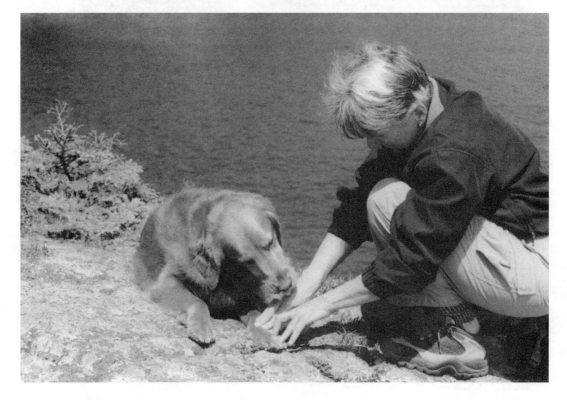

Acknowledgments

Thanks to all of the people who so generously agreed to be a part of this project. This is their way of giving you, the reader, a taste of what is possible through the healing powers of Rolfing® Structural Integration.

I want to thank Carrie Voyles, a medical transcriber, who carefully and accurately transcribed all the interviews I conducted. I am also appreciative of her initial editing of most of this book.

I am deeply filled with gratitude to my friend and Rolfing SI colleague, Marilyn Beech, for coming into this project at a crucial moment in the evolution of this book. We have shared the path and mission of this Rolfing SI work and she has been an integral part of my history. Marilyn served as my final editor, writer (when restructuring was called for), and guide in the final weaving of bringing this book project to completion. She has also been a great advisor in steering this book into final edited form.

I am appreciative to my literary agent, book consultant, and friend, Laurie Harper, for always watching my back and guiding me to the right publisher for this book. Her deep knowledge and experience in the publishing world has kept me on track so I could clearly accomplish the outcome I desired to produce.

A big thank you to Judy Gilats, of Peregrine Graphics Services, for her meticulous and artistic layout of this book. She has more than accomplished her plan to "exceed" my expectations. I applaud you for your artistry, work ethic, and giving me your best.

There are countless people who also contributed their time and energy with this book. A huge thank you to Paul Schurke, Wintergreen Dogsled Lodge, for reading the manuscript, writing the foreword, and providing a quote for the back cover.

To Dr. Julie Wilson, Associate Professor with the University of Minnesota, The College of Veterinary Medicine, for inviting me into her world to rehab a young colt, doing presentations to vet students, and for collaborating in this book with a story and a book review.

I am grateful to MaryBeth Garrigan, Program Director at the National Eagle Center (2000–2009) for allowing me to work with four different eagles over a two and one-half year period of time and for staying after hours many Fridays so that I could do my rehabilitation with the eagles. I am also indebted to Scott Mehus, Education Director; Bridget Beforg, Program Specialist; and to Volunteer Eagle handlers, Dennis and Dottie Flint, who also stayed many Friday nights.

I'm indebted to Dr. Allen Schoen for his early recognition and support of my work, for his input with this manuscript, and his deep understanding and appreciation of the power of Rolfing® SI.

Many others assisted me with a variety of services. I am most appreciative of my colleague Stephen Evanko who graciously provided me with the fascia photos. Cole Stewart, Assistant Manager of PROEX who has developed hundreds of my photographs, helping me whenever technical help was needed. Bev Asher and Celeste Mazur for accompanying me to Ely, Minnesota, and assisting me with the sled dogs. Cindy Due has been an angel in my life giving me technical help, computer assistance, and secretarial help when I was in a pinch. Carolyn Alfonso, Grif Sadow, Celeste Mazur, and Bill Slobotski for all their final-hour creative and technical assistance, as well as Celeste for proofing the manuscript.

A big thank you also goes out to my team at Mill City Press who took this project to the final book production.

About the Author

Throughout **BRIAH ANSON**'s life she has been a pioneer. Her key strength is her breadth of experience with integrated care modalities coupled with her commitment to enriching every client, person, or animal with whom she works.

This calling began in Costa Rica where Briah grew up pursuing and becoming a highly trained athlete, ballet dancer, and nationally competitive swimmer, golfer (four-time Junior National Golf Champion of Costa Rica) and tennis player. At age seventeen, she set the Costa Rican women's Olympic javelin record.

Today, Briah is a Certified Advanced Rolfer™ and Rolf Movement® Practitioner with over thirty years of experience. In addition to writing and teaching engagements, she maintains a private practice in St. Paul, Minnesota.

She is the author and publisher of *Rolfing®: Stories of Personal Empowerment* (1991; 1992, Heartland Personal Growth Press). She copublished the same book with North Atlantic Books in 1998. She also produced and directed the video entitled *Growing Right with Rolfing®*, 1996, a documentary featuring her work with children under the age of four.

In 1968 Briah received her BA degree from Oakland University and an MA in Counseling and College Student Personnel from Pennsylvania State University in 1971. She was a member of the Dean of Students' staff at Penn State, Colorado College, and the University of Minnesota, Morris, in the late 1960s and 1970s.

In 1979 she became one of the earliest pioneers in Rolfing® SI for animals and over the next twelve years produced five educational videos on that work. Briah moved to Kansas City in 1979, where she developed her practice as a Rolfer™ and where she cofounded Heartland Personal

Growth Center, and then founded Heartland Rolfing® Associates in 1997. In July of 1998, Briah moved to the Twin Cities where she established Rolfing® and Healing Arts Associates and currently has a private practice.

Continuing her evolution as a healer, Briah completed her training and certification in 2001 as a practitioner of Frequencies of Brilliance—a form of energetic body work—with Christine Day. Briah has dedicated herself to the exploration and interface of how Rolfing and the Frequencies of Brilliance alter both the structure of her clients as well as their emerging consciousness. To date, she has received twelve stages of the Frequencies of Brilliance training.

Briah is a member of the Rolf Institute® of Structural Integration, the International Association of Structural Integrators®, and serves on the Board of Directors of the Northwestern Academy of Homeopathy in Minneapolis, Minnesota.

www.rolfing-briahanson.com

Basil (Wyndcrest Grand Illusion)
"Messenger of Peace"
Courtesy of Jill Rivard

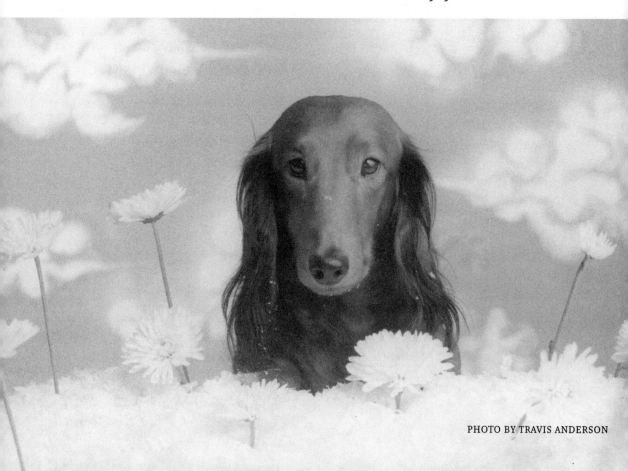

PHOTO BY TRAVIS ANDERSON